Ginger Sullivan

the Honeymooner's Cookbook

52 weeks of food and sex

For food lovers who want to cook up a lasting love affair

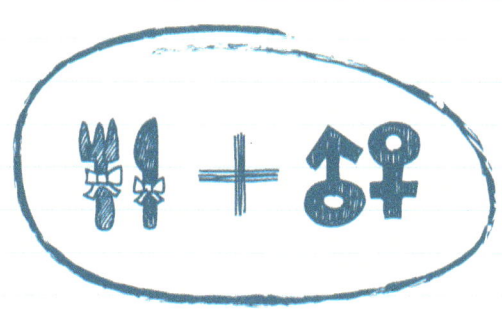

Published in 2015 by H&A
© 2015 H&A

This book is strictly for readers aged 18 years and over. All rights reserved. No part of this publication may be reproduced, stored in a retrieval system or transmitted in any form or by any means, without the express, written permission of the publisher. The information, content and materials published in this book, including without limitation, text and graphics are provided on an "as-is" basis. The Proprietor makes no representations or warranties of any kind, express or implied, as to the accuracy, correctness or completeness of the information, contents, materials, products, services included in this book. This book is designed to be humorous and entertaining and by no means aims to replace guidance obtained from professional advice. In no event shall the author or H&A be liable for any direct, indirect, punitive, incidental, special or consequential damages arising out of or in any way connected with the use of this material.

First published 2015

ISBN: 978-0-620-66954-2

Editor: Bethany Reed
Proofreader: Amalia Christoforou
Book and Cover Design by: Samantha Rowles
Typesetting and Layout by: Samantha Rowles
Illustrations: Johann Strauss

H&A
Postnet Suite 749
Private Bag X153
Bryanston
Republic of South Africa

Contents

Early-morning Nookie — 9 — Breakfast

The Push Start	10	great-start scrambled egg
The Morning Glory	12	zinger smoothie
The Helicopter	14	mile-high omelette
The Personal Trainer	16	health sundae
The Shaven Haven	18	sweet patties
The Twister	20	cinnamon twists
The See-Saw	22	playful flapjacks
The Comfort Zone	24	cosy egg nests
The Couch Potato	26	dirty little mince pies

Between Bites — 29 — Light Snacks

The Water Quickie	30	boisterous oysters
The Pamper Party	32	cheat pizza
The Foot Fettish	34	tommy-toe tomato salad
The Porno	36	potent panini
The Artist	38	baked camembert 2 die 4
The Love Birds	40	duo terrine
The Channel Hog	42	bacon butty
The Extreme Makeover	44	mix-it-up meze
The Lotus Surprise	46	wanton noodles
The Hole In One	48	devilish hearts
The Secret	50	macho gazpacho
The Sneaky Bastard	52	quickie turkey sandwich
The Sun Goddess	54	moist and fiery salmon
The Dragon Tamer	58	silky tomato soup
The Free Ride	60	tantalising tagliolini
The Hard Yards	62	forking fantastic toasties

NIGHT-TIME RENDEZVOUS 65 DINNER

The Duet	66	fish with rösti
The Cheerleader	68	burger deluxe
The Wrestler	70	fancy-pants fillet
The Tango	72	drop-your-panties gnocchi
The Back Flip	74	sweet and supple chick
The Crack Filler	76	beef shank bone
The Side Saddle	78	lusty langoustines
The Star Gazer	80	heavenly thighs
The Peeping Tom	82	surreal casserole
The Opera	84	velvety tagliatelle
The Windy Shaft	86	left-over wine
The Naughty Nurse	88	hot stuff lamb
The Skipper	90	rocking kabeljou
The Grower	92	beefy wellies
The Greek Dip	94	greek-style kebabs
The Swinger	96	succulent plum fillet

HAPPY ENDINGS 99 DESSERT

The Bungee Jumper	100	drunken pavlova
The Tattoo	102	seductive marshmallows
The Ice Dancer	104	frozen kahlua cake
The Learner Driver	106	travelling chocolate pots
The Babymaker	108	celebration jelly
The Multi-Tasker	110	coconut pleasure
The Party Quickie	112	melt-in-mouth meringue
The Virgin	114	pop-the-cherry pie
The Balancing Act	116	spicy custard

*Let's be honest,
you need just 50 recipes.*

*You won't leave the bedroom
for the first two weeks.*

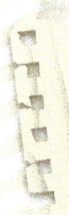

Set the mood by laying a table and always use your best tableware.

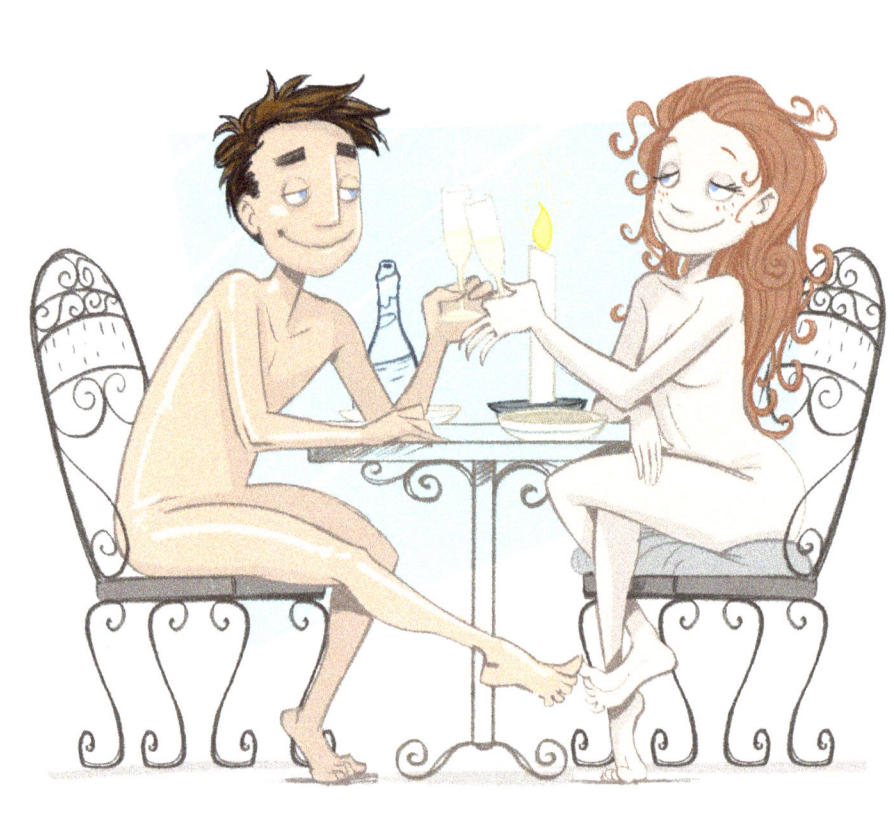

Pick a position and whet your appetite.

Notes

Breakfast

early-morning nookie

The Push Start

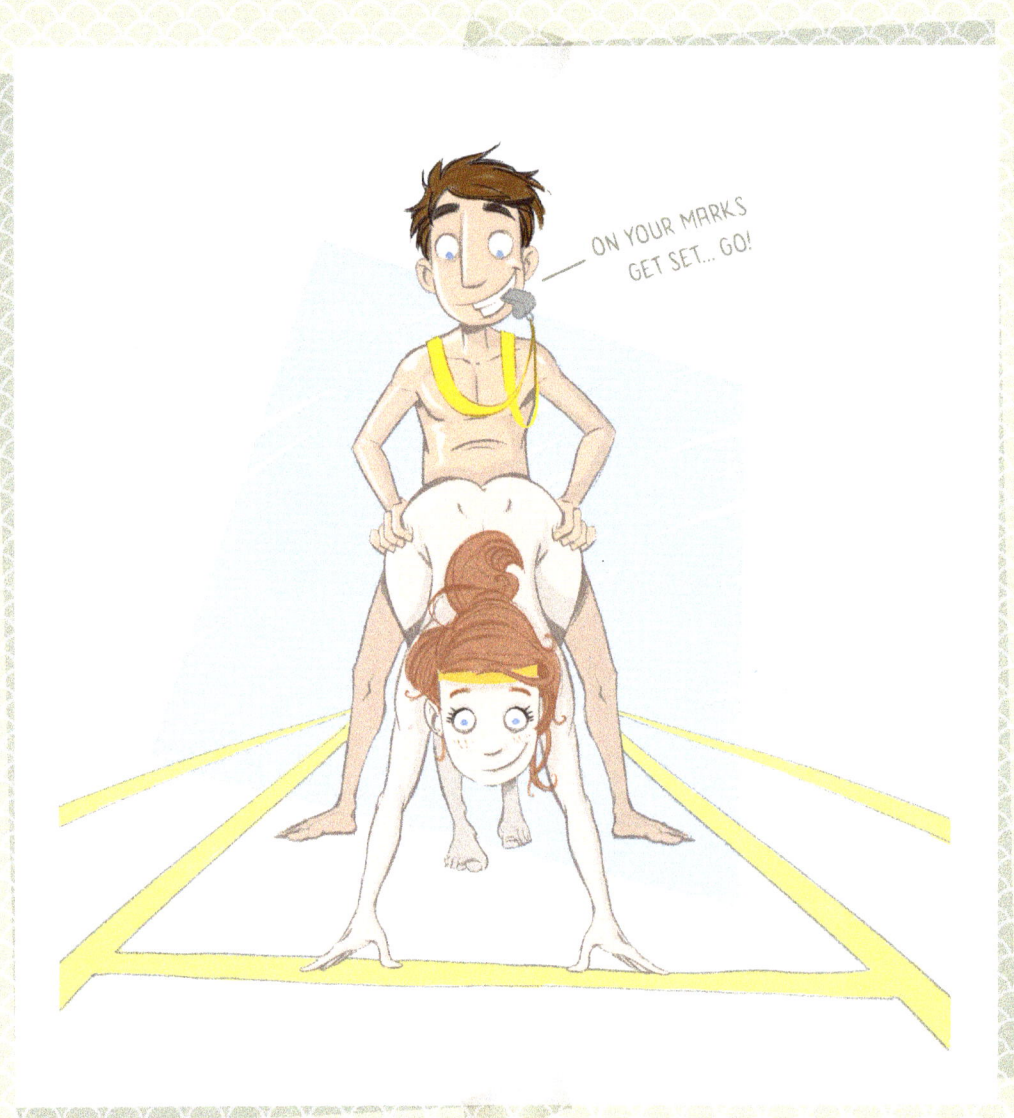

great-start scrambled egg

easy
15 min

- 4 eggs
- knob of butter
- ¼ cup parmesan cheese, finely grated
- 100g salmon ribbons, sliced
- 1 tbsp chives, chopped, for garnishing
- black pepper

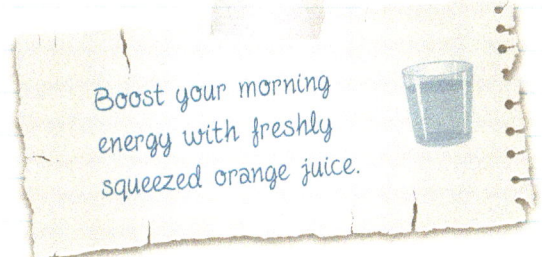

Boost your morning energy with freshly squeezed orange juice.

Crack the eggs into a jug and lightly whisk. Bring a pan to medium heat and add the butter. When the butter has melted, spread it around the pan and pour in the egg. Stir gently with a wooden spoon but remove the eggs from the heat just before they are ready because they will continue to cook. Transfer the eggs to a small serving dish and move to a warming tray. Sprinkle a thin layer of cheese over the egg. Arrange the salmon over the cheese, garnish with chives and season. Serve with lightly buttered toast.

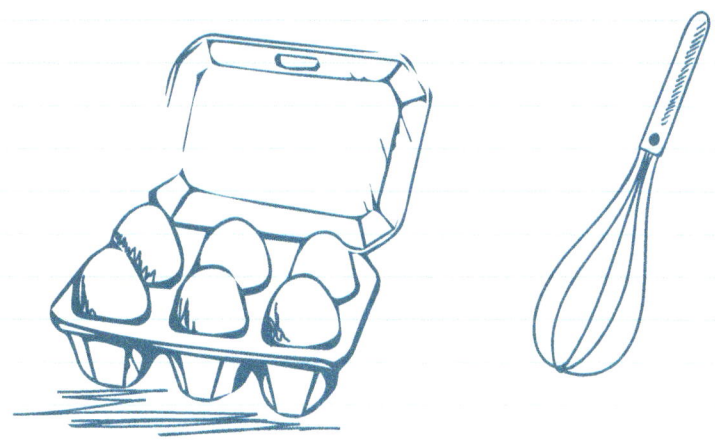

The Morning Glory

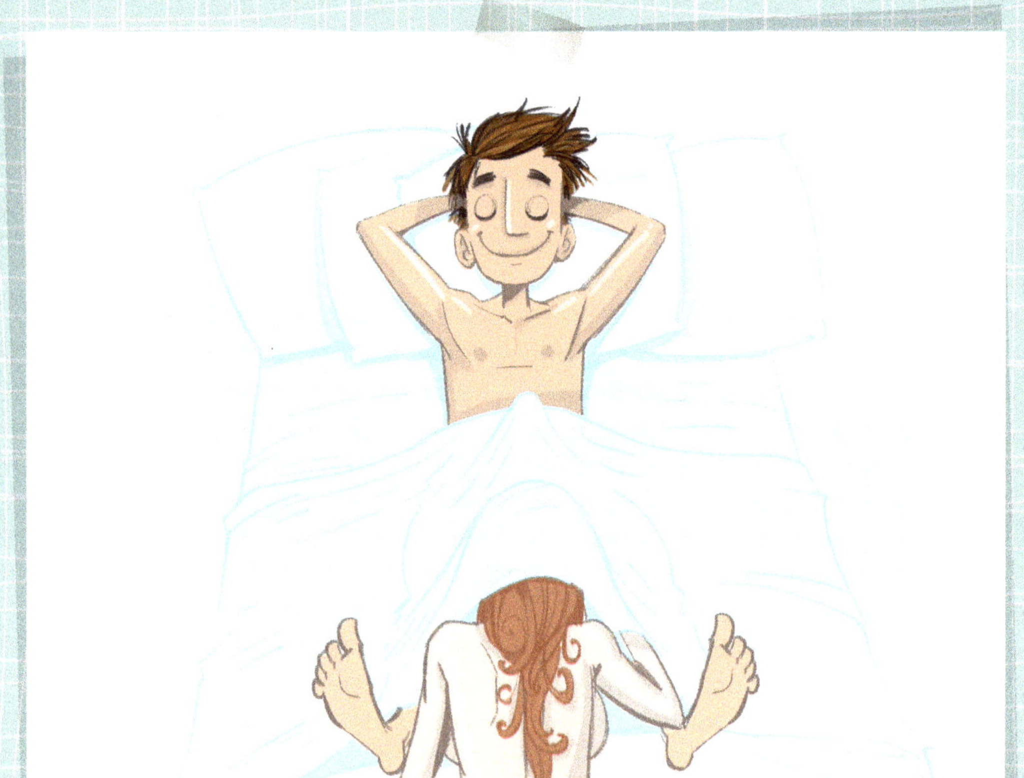

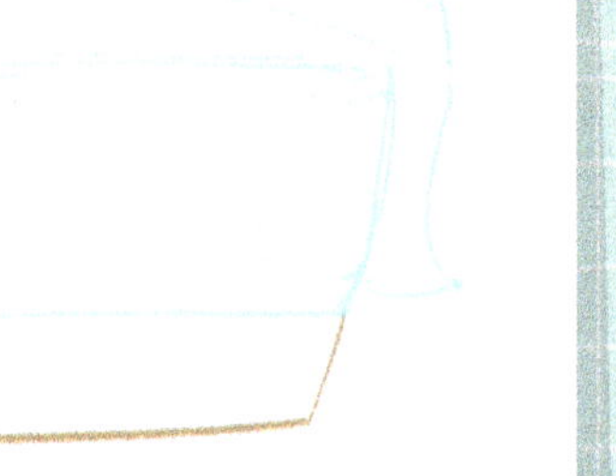

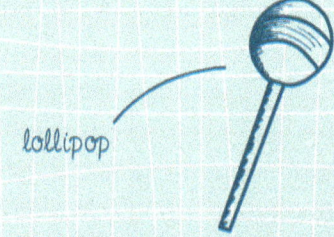

lollipop

zinger smoothie

 easy

 20 min

- 4 green apples, cored and peeled
- 4 pears, cored and peeled
- 1 finger ginger root, peeled and grated
- 6 sprigs fresh mint, leaves picked
- 1 tbsp fresh lime juice
- 1 lime, sliced

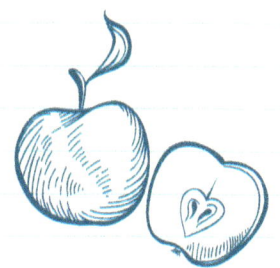
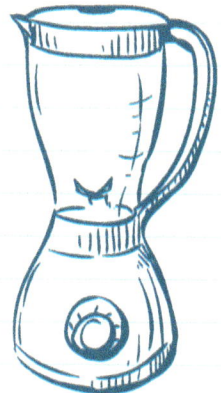

Steam the apples and pears for 10 minutes or until soft. Allow to cool. Put the fruit, ginger, mint and lime juice into a blender, and whizz until smooth.

Add 1 cup of crushed ice and whizz for an additional 3 seconds. Pour into tall glasses and garnish with the lime. Serve with a few slices of brown toast, butter and preserves.

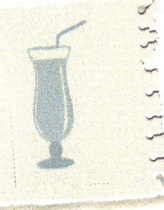

Trigger your sexual prowess with a few sips of this zinger ginger smoothie, before going to wake your partner.

The Helicopter

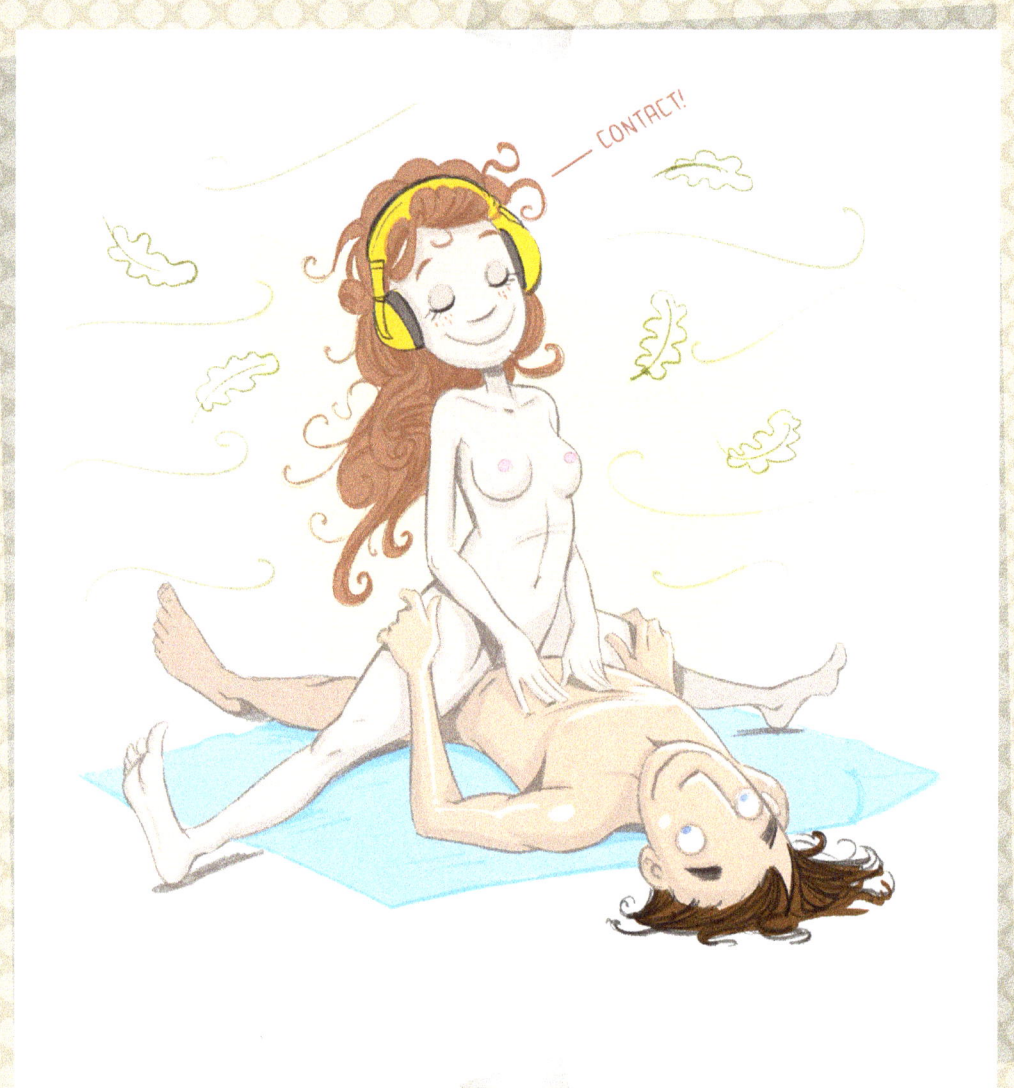

mile-high omelette

easy

25 min

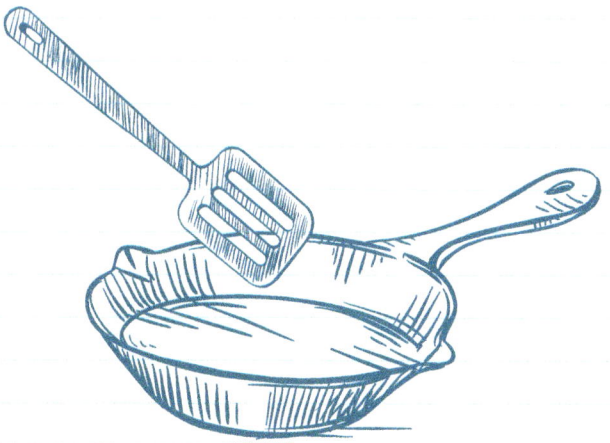

- 2 handfuls baby spinach
- olive oil
- 6 eggs, lightly beaten
- ½ cup feta
- handful sun-dried tomatoes, coarsely chopped
- salt and pepper
- 1 avocado, peeled and sliced
- 1 lemon, quartered
- handful fresh baby rocket

Lightly steam the spinach until just wilted, squeeze out the excess water and slice it into ribbons. Set aside.

Heat a medium-sized non-stick pan and lightly grease with a little olive oil. Pour in half the egg, swirling over the base of the pan. Cook until the base is set and the top is still runny. Crumble the feta over the runny section and arrange the sun-dried tomatoes and spinach over the feta. Season and then use an egg-lifter to carefully fold the sides over the filling. Cook for an additional minute. Repeat with the remaining egg. Serve with the slices of avocado and garnish with lemon and rocket.

Recommended:
Some believe peppery rocket will boost your libido... that's worth a try! Crack open a dry Methode Cap Classique to magnify the mood.

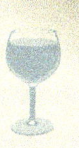

The Personal Trainer

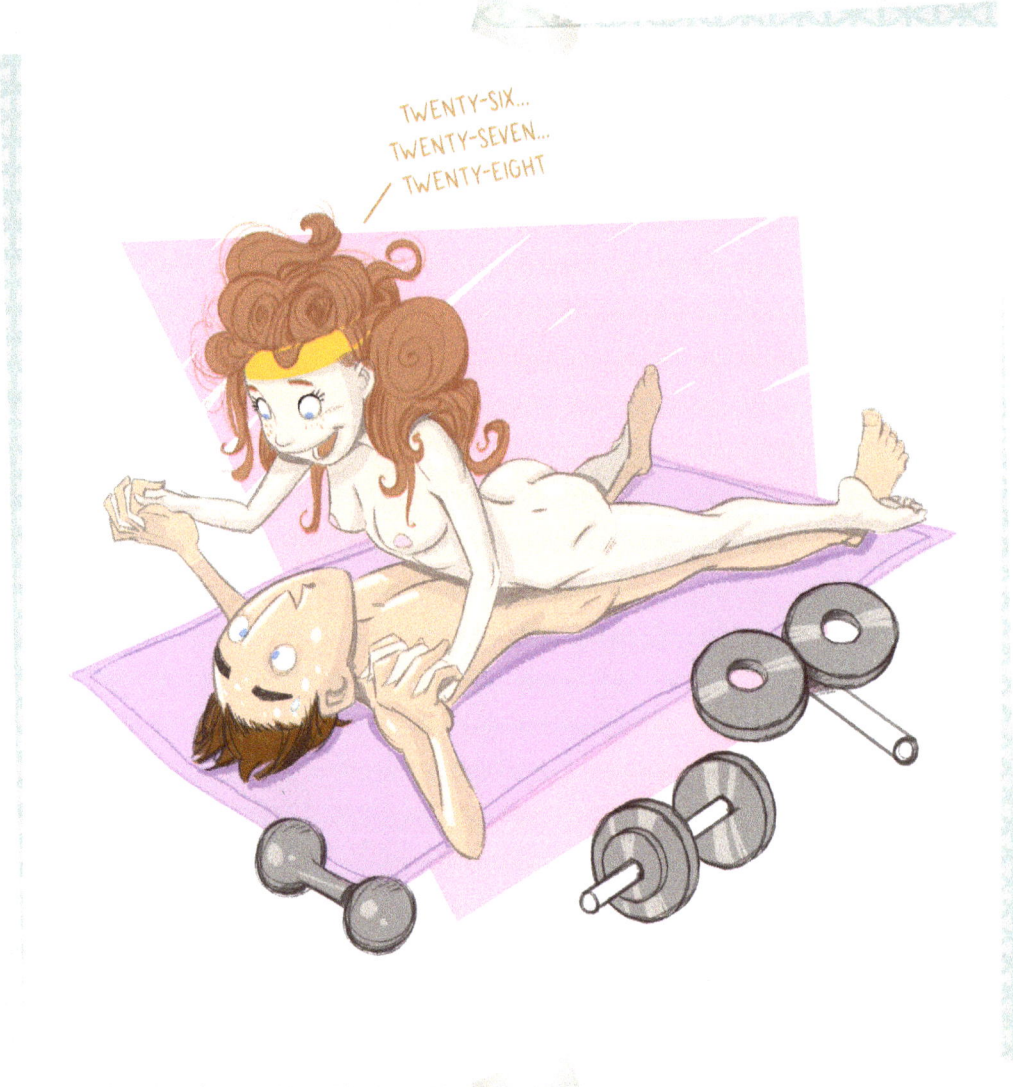

health sundae

easy

10 min

- 1 cup toasted muesli
- 1 small papaya, peeled and cubed
- 2 cups double cream yogurt
- handful flaked almonds, toasted
- honey
- sprig fresh mint

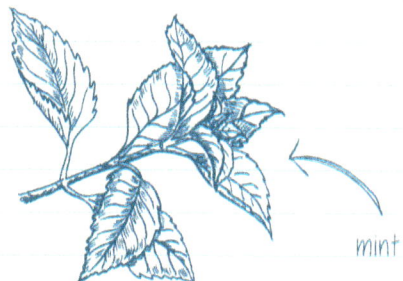
mint

Divide the muesli into two sundae glasses. Put the papaya cubes on top of the muesli and smother with yogurt. Sprinkle over the almonds, drizzle with honey and finish off with a sprig of mint.

Trickle a little honey over your partner for a second delight.

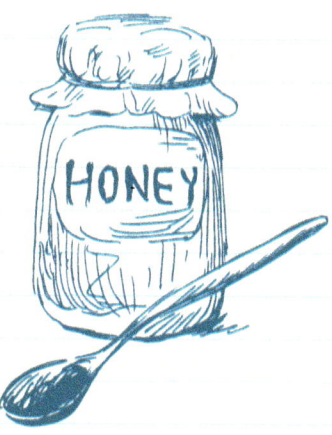

The Shaven Haven

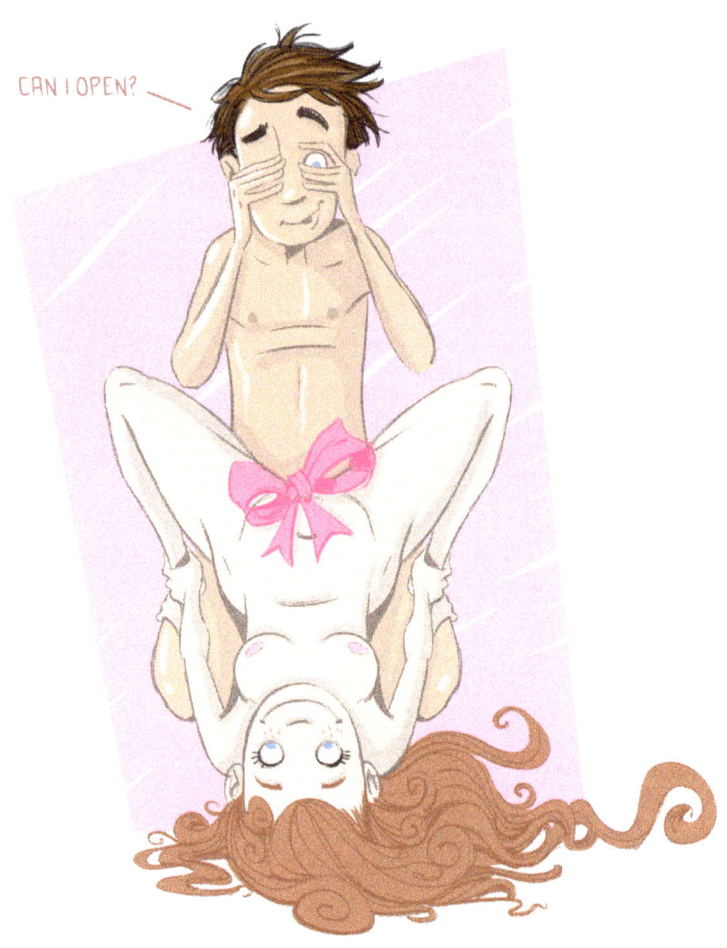

Yummy with a steaming shot of espresso...

sweet patties

a little effort

30 min

- 1 sweet potato, sliced
- sprig fresh rosemary, finely chopped
- sprig fresh thyme, finely chopped
- 8 cherry tomatoes, halved
- olive oil
- 1 cup boerenkaas cheese, finely grated
- 2 eggs
- 1 tbsp white wine vinegar
- salt and pepper
- dash balsamic vinegar
- sprig thyme, for garnishing

Cook the sweet potato in a microwave oven for 5 minutes and allow to cool slightly. Chop it up and mix in the herbs. Take large spoonfuls of the mixture and flatten them into patties. Place the patties on a greased baking tray and grill until golden brown. Drizzle the tomatoes with oil and pop into the oven at the same time as the patties, to grill until soft. Sprinkle the cheese on patties and put the patties back under the grill until the cheese is just melted. Poach the eggs and serve them on top of the patties with the tomatoes arranged around the plate. Season and add an attractive drizzle of balsamic vinegar and thyme leaves.

Tip:
To poach eggs, fill ¾ of a pan with water and bring to the boil. Add the vinegar and reduce the heat until it simmers. Crack one egg at a time into a cup and carefully drop it into the water. Cook for a few minutes until the white of the egg has set but the yolk is still runny. Scoop the eggs from the water and serve.

THE TWISTER

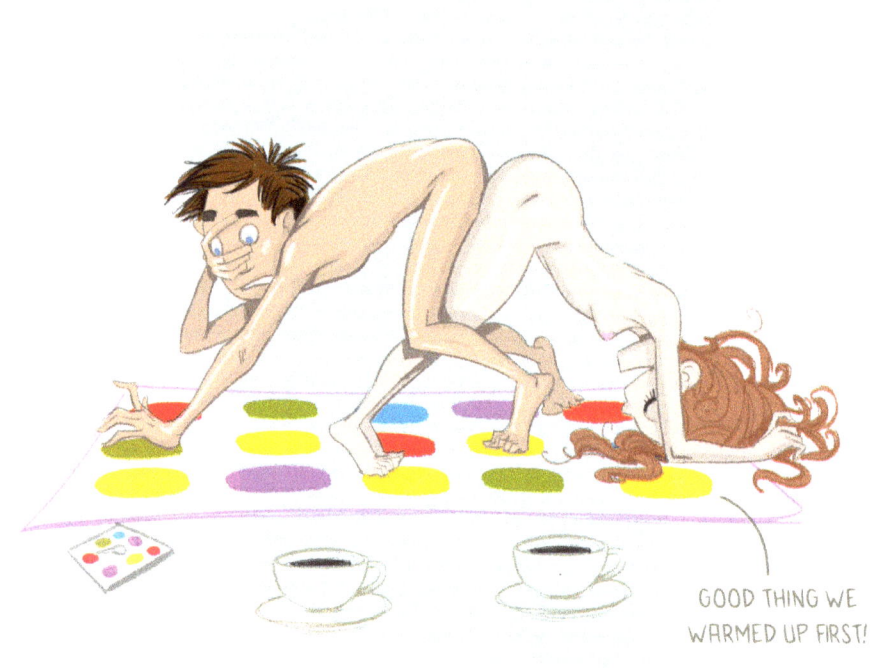

GOOD THING WE WARMED UP FIRST!

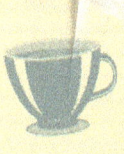

You will go nuts for these pastries served with a couple of cappuccinos.

cinnamon twists

a lot of effort

\> 60 min

PASTRY
- 5g instant dry yeast
- ¼ cup warm water
- ½ cup buttermilk
- 2 tbsp unsalted butter, softened
- 1 egg
- 1 tbsp brown sugar
- pinch of salt
- ¼ tsp bicarbonate of soda
- 2 cups cake flour, sifted
- non-stick spray, for greasing

FILLING
- 1 tbsp unsalted butter, melted
- ¼ cup brown sugar
- ½ tsp ground cinnamon
- ¼ cup raw pecan nuts, peeled and chopped

Use grated marzipan and flaked almonds for an alternative filling.

ICING
- ½ cup icing sugar
- knob of butter, melted
- 3 tbsp hot water
- 1 vanilla pod, seeds removed

Dissolve the yeast in warm water. In a mixing bowl combine the yeast, buttermilk, butter, egg, sugar, salt, bicarbonate of soda and flour, stirring well to form a dough. Move the dough to a clean surface, sprinkle with flour and knead the dough until it is smooth. Grease a large bowl with non-stick spray and put the dough in the bowl. Cover the bowl with a cloth and allow to rise in warm place. When the dough has doubled in size, move it to a clean surface dusted with flour and roll it out into a rectangle, about 4mm thick.

Just before starting the filling, brush the dough with melted butter. Combine the sugar and cinnamon and sprinkle it evenly over the melted butter. Sprinkle the nuts over half of the pastry and then fold it to make a rectangle. Pinch the edges closed and then cut into 3cm strips. Twist each strip 3 to 5 times and place it on a greased baking tray far enough apart to allow for expansion. Cover with a cloth and allow to rise in a warm place. When it has doubled in size, bake at 190°C for 15 minutes or until golden brown.

To make the icing, whisk together the icing sugar, butter, water and vanilla seeds. Move the twists to a cooling rack and drizzle with the glaze while they are still warm.

The See-Saw

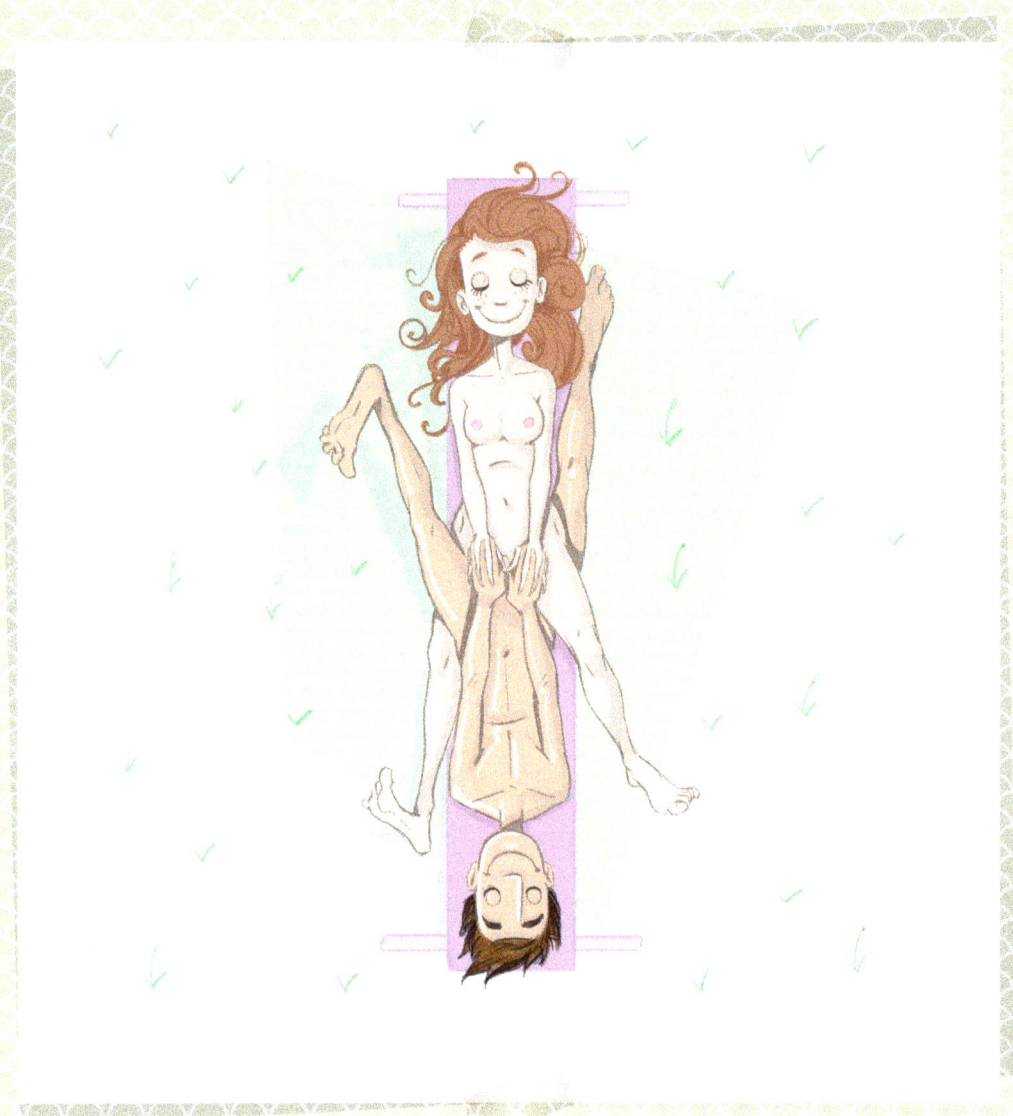

playful flapjacks

easy
25 min

- 1 cup self-raising flour
- 1 cup milk
- 1 large egg
- pinch of salt
- unsalted butter, for frying
- 100g mascarpone
- ½ cup strawberries, stalks removed and quartered
- 2 tbsp flaked almonds, toasted
- honey, for drizzling

Combine the flour, milk, egg and salt in a mixing bowl, and mix well with an electric beater until smooth.

Bring a heavy-based pan to a medium heat and add a knob of butter. When the butter has melted, spoon the batter into the pan using a ladle, so that you have about four flapjacks cooking at one time. Cook until you see little bubbles appearing on top and the bottom is starting to turn golden. Turn over the flapjacks to brown the other side and then transfer them to a dish on a warming tray. Repeat until all the flapjacks are cooked, cleaning the pan with a paper towel between each batch.

To serve, spread a generous layer of mascarpone over each flapjack. Top with the strawberries, almonds and a drizzle of honey and serve with a chilled smoothie.

Recommended:
Blend a banana, ½ cup orange juice, ice and a handful of mixed berries to make a smoothie. Pour into a champagne flute, pop in a straw and garnish with a slice of orange.

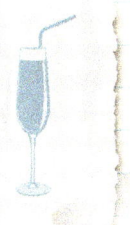

The Comfort Zone

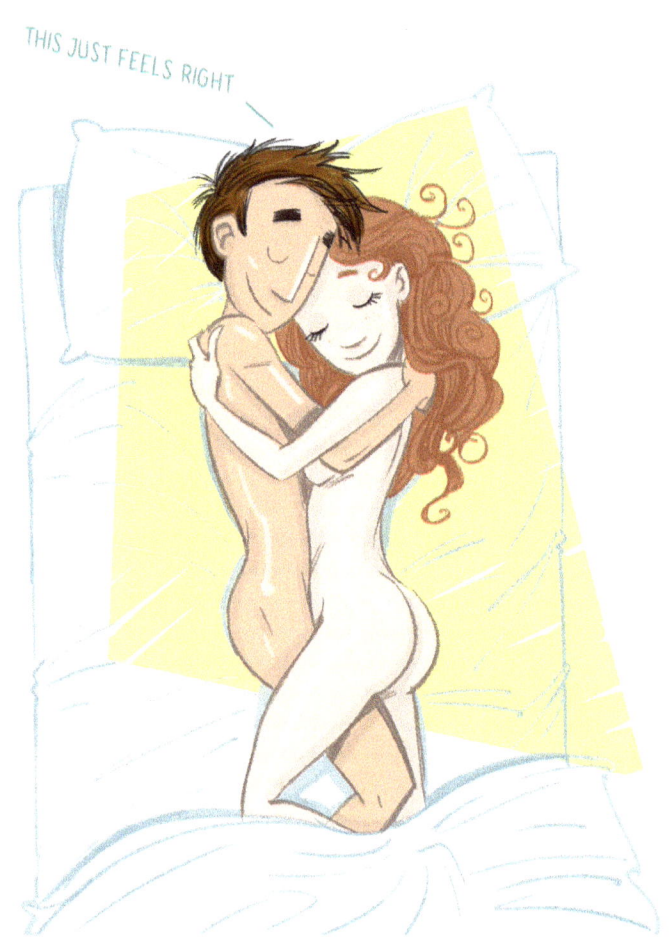

cosy egg nests

a little effort

30 min

- 1 packet ready-made puff pastry, defrosted
- knob of butter
- handful portobello mushrooms, sliced
- sprig fresh thyme, leaves picked
- 6 rosa tomatoes, sliced
- 2 small chipolata sausages, cooked and sliced
- 2 eggs
- salt and pepper
- 2 tbsp gruyere cheese, grated
- sprig fresh basil, for garnishing

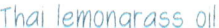

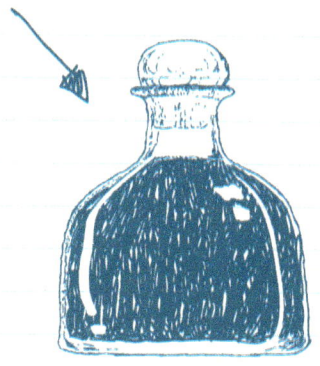

Thai lemongrass oil

Warm up some massage oil and explore each other.

Lightly grease 2 cups in a muffin pan. Using a large cookie cutter, cut out two circles from the pastry. Lay the pastry in the tray and using a fork, prick a few holes in the bottom. Heat the butter in a pan and fry the mushrooms and thyme until golden. Add the tomatoes and cook just enough to soften. Divide the mushrooms, tomatoes and sausage between the two muffins. Crack an egg into each one, and season. Bake for 15 minutes at 200°C. Sprinkle the cheese on top, and bake for an additional 5 minutes until the pastry is golden. Allow to cool a little before taking out the pan. Garnish with basil. Double the filling ingredients to make 4 muffins.

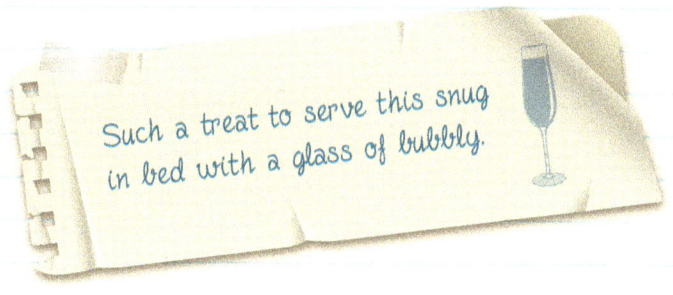

Such a treat to serve this snug in bed with a glass of bubbly.

The Couch Potato

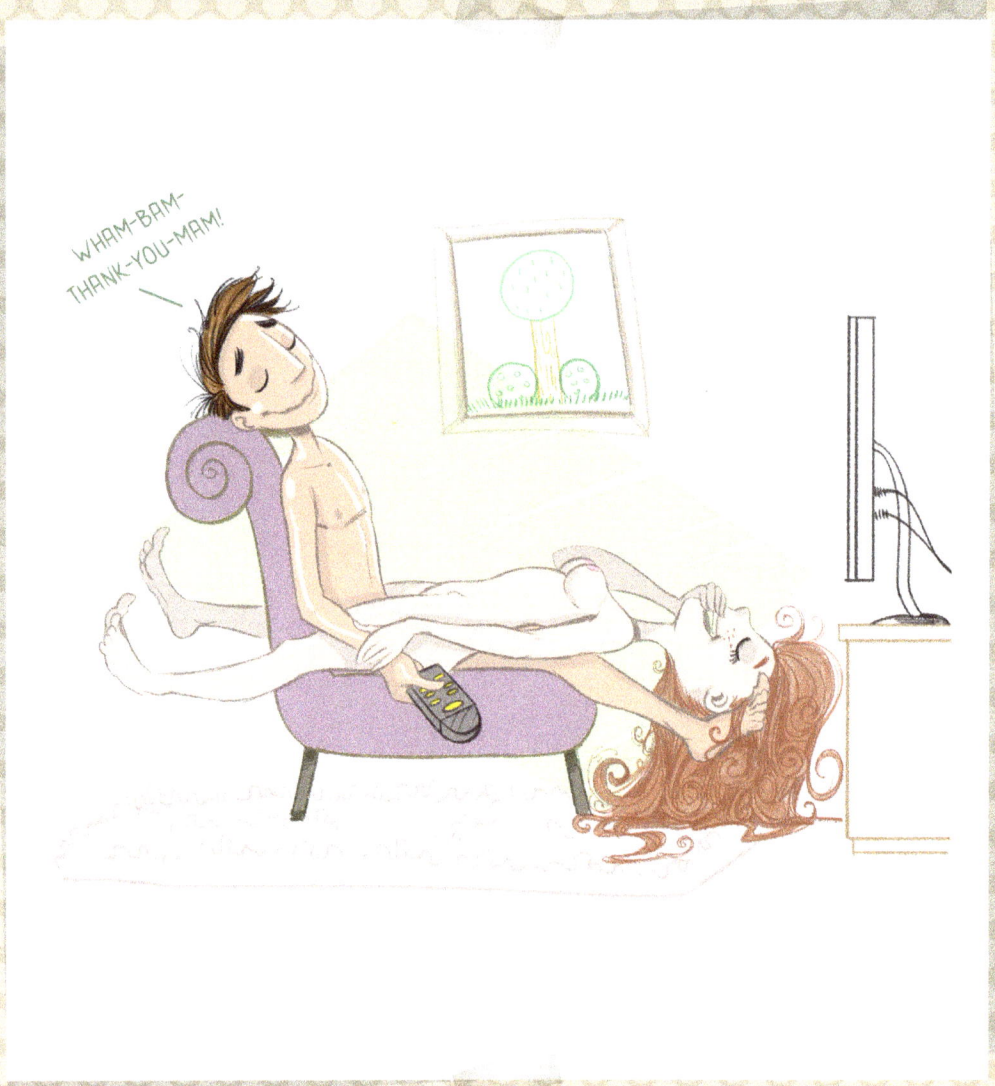

dirty little mince pies

easy
10 min

- ½ cup double thick cream
- 4 mince pies
- pinch cinnamon
- good whisky, preferably peaty

Warm the pies and drop a dollop of cream next to them. Sprinkle a little cinnamon onto the cream and drizzle with a dash of whisky.

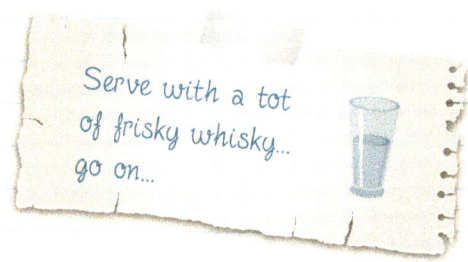

Serve with a tot of frisky whisky... go on...

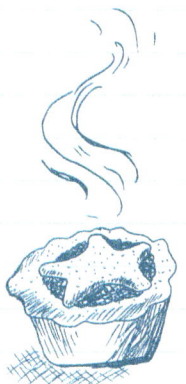

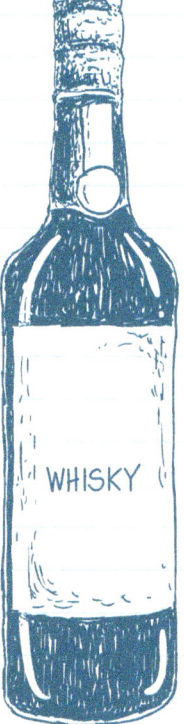

Perfect for when you feel lethargic and don't want to cook. Keep a dozen store-bought mince pies in your freezer for times like these. It's quick and dirty, just the way your partner likes it.

Notes

Light Snacks

between bites

The Water Quickie

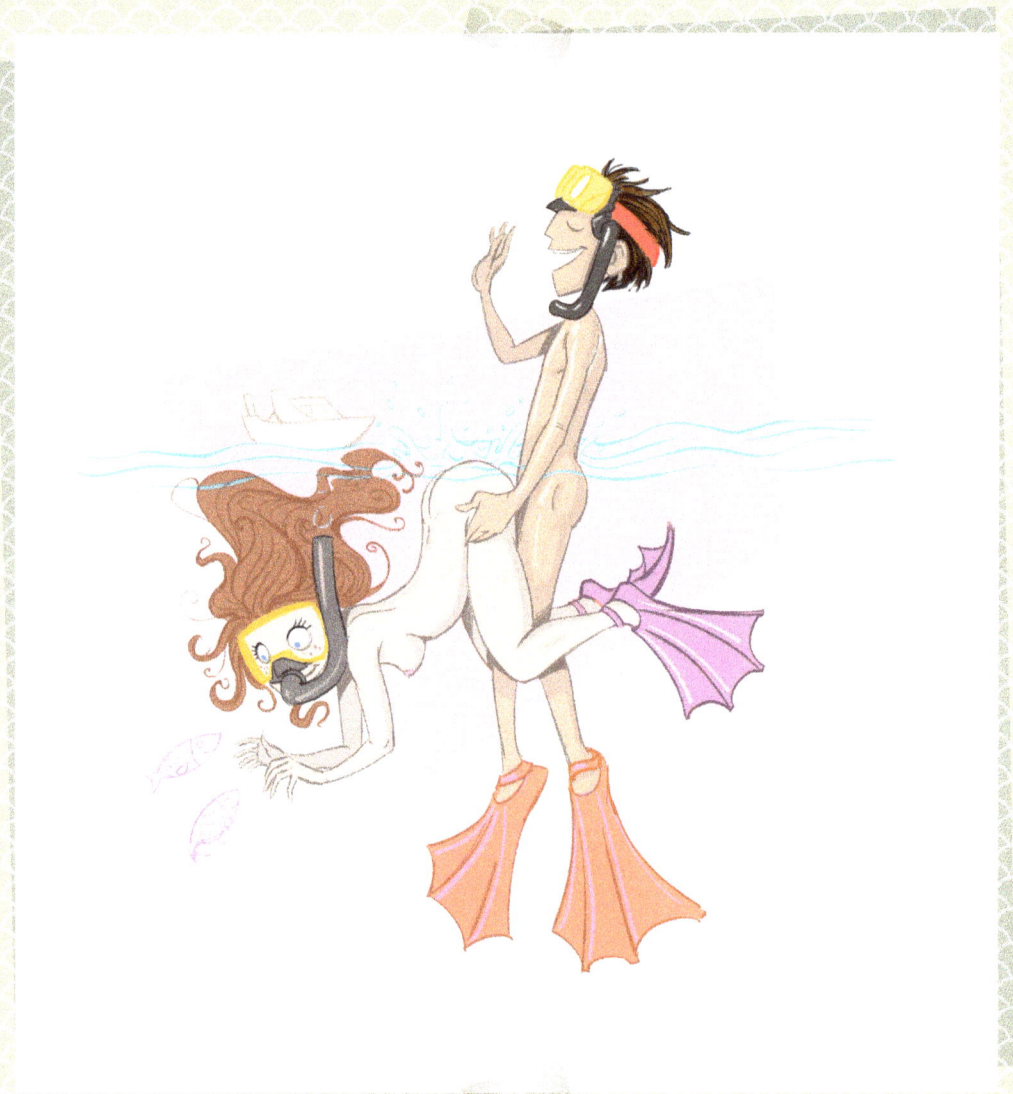

Crank up the testosterone with this quick dish.

boisterous oysters

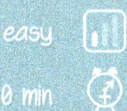

easy
10 min

- 12 oysters, top shell removed
- 4 lemon wedges
- tabasco sauce
- black pepper

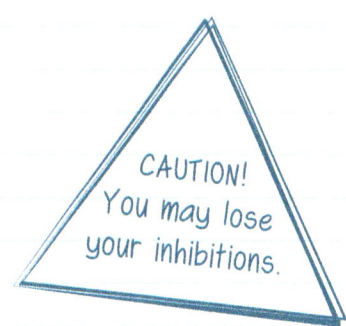

CAUTION! You may lose your inhibitions.

If you have a good fishmonger close by, pick up some fresh oysters and take them home to prepare.

Arrange the oysters on a platter over a bed of crushed ice. Squeeze lemon juice over each oyster, give it a dash of tabasco and season.

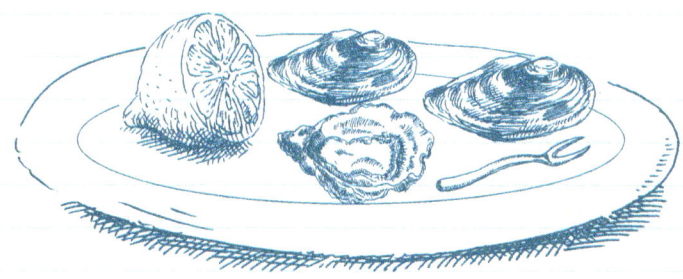

Recommended:
Since you are already splashing out on oysters, go all the way and pair it with a vintage Champagne.

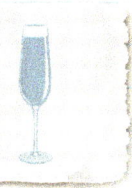

The Pamper Party

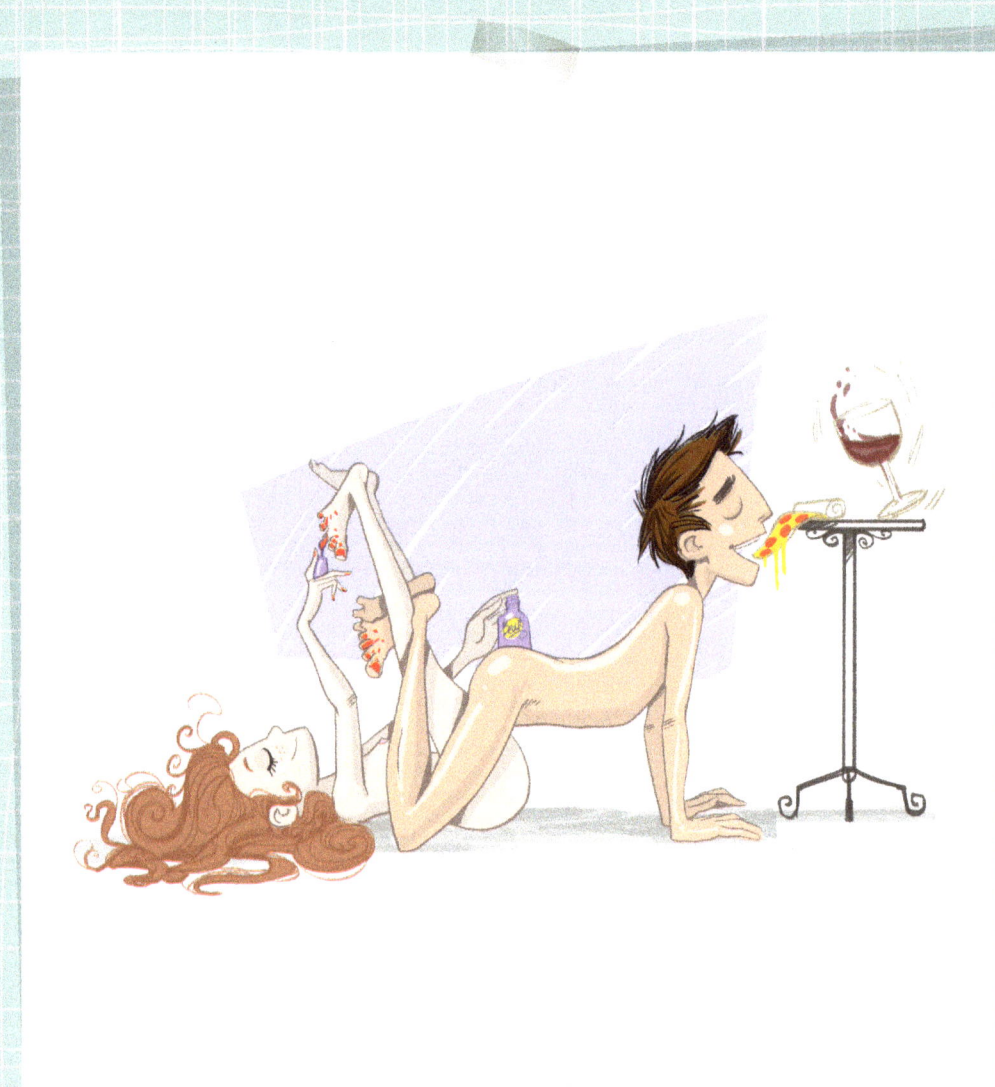

cheat pizza

a little effort
30 min

- 1 packet ready-made puff pastry, defrosted
- 1 egg, beaten
- 2 tbsp olive tapenade
- 1½ cups mozzarella, grated
- ¼ cup parmesan, finely grated
- handful basil leaves, chopped
- sprig fresh thyme, leaves picked
- ground black pepper
- ½ cup rosa tomatoes, halved
- 2 slices parma ham, cut into strips
- handful baby rocket leaves

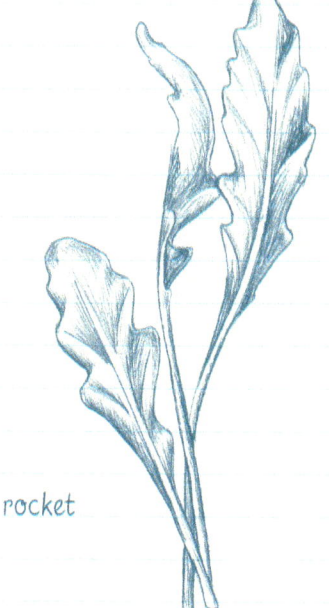

rocket

Lay the pastry out on a baking tray lined with wax paper. Using a fork prick a few holes in the base. Brush the egg to make a 2cm-thick frame around the pastry. Smear the tapenade evenly over the pastry keeping to the inside of the frame. In a bowl, mix the cheese and herbs and then sprinkle the cheese mixture over the tapenade and season. Top with the tomatoes and ham. Pop in the oven for 20 minutes at 200°C until the pastry is golden and cheese beautifully melted. Allow to rest for a few minutes before slicing. Garnish with rocket leaves and serve.

Recommended:
A chocolate Pinotage is a delightful companion to this snack.

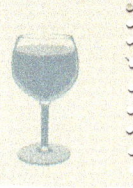

THE FOOT FETTISH

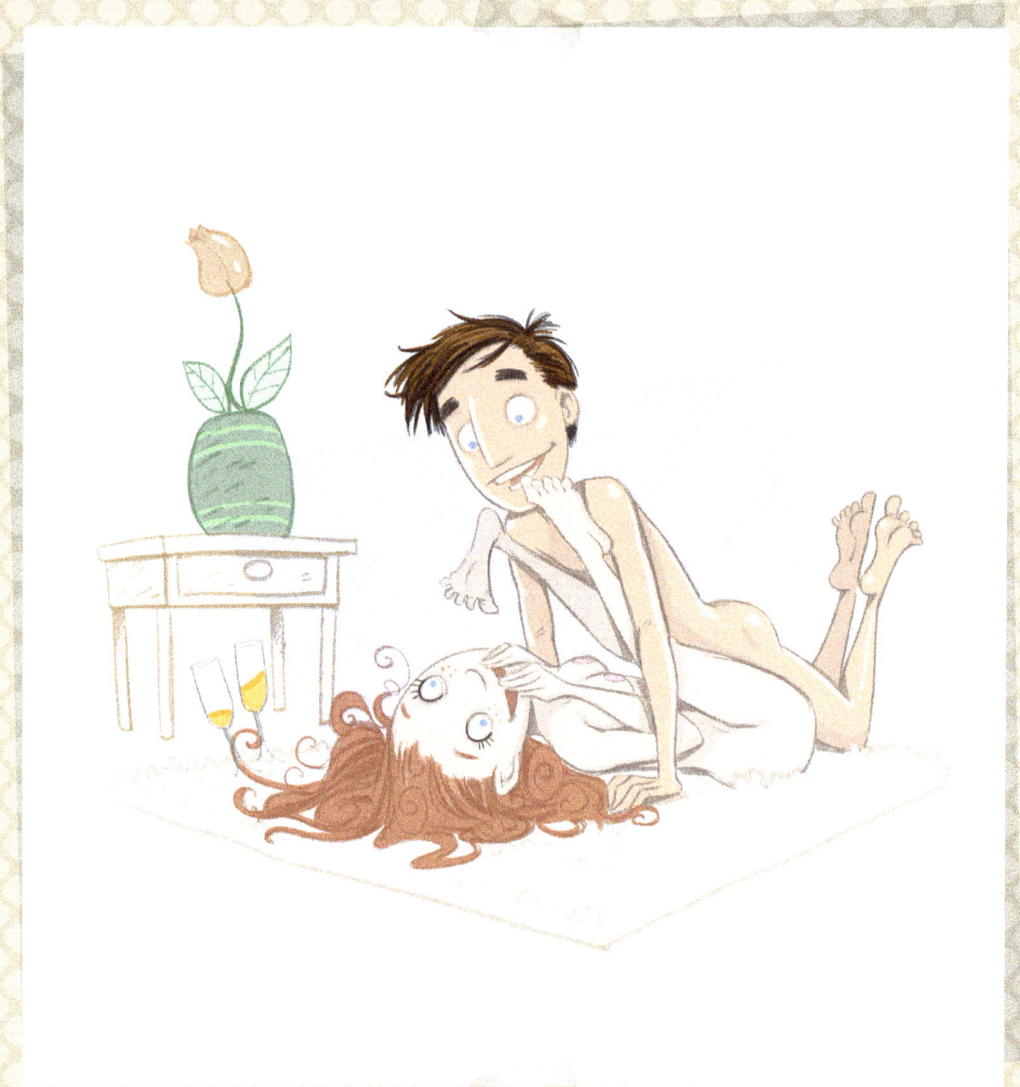

34

tommy-toe tomato salad

easy
20 min

- ¼ cup pine nuts
- 3 cups cherry tomatoes, halved
- ¼ cup large black olives, pitted and halved
- ½ cup buffalo mozzarella balls, shredded
- good-quality olive oil, for drizzling
- handful fresh basil, leaves picked
- salt and pepper
- 4 thick slices crusty bread
- good-quality butter
- balsamic vinegar, for drizzling

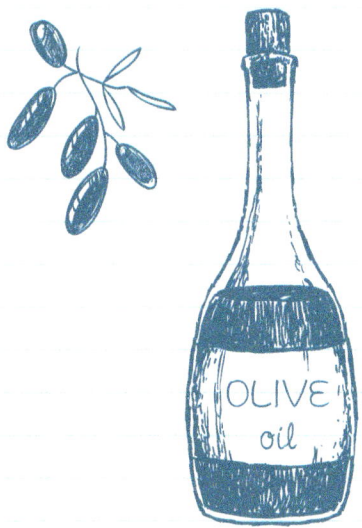

Bring a non-stick pan to a medium heat, and lightly toast the nuts until golden brown, tossing frequently. Set aside to cool.

Add the tomatoes, olives, nuts and cheese to a mixing bowl and toss well. Drizzle with olive oil and toss again to coat the salad. Garnish with the basil and season to taste. Serve alongside warm, generously-buttered bread drizzled with balsamic vinegar.

Recommended:
In-between the nibbling, enjoy a flute of chilled sparkling Rosé wine.

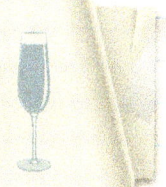

The Porno

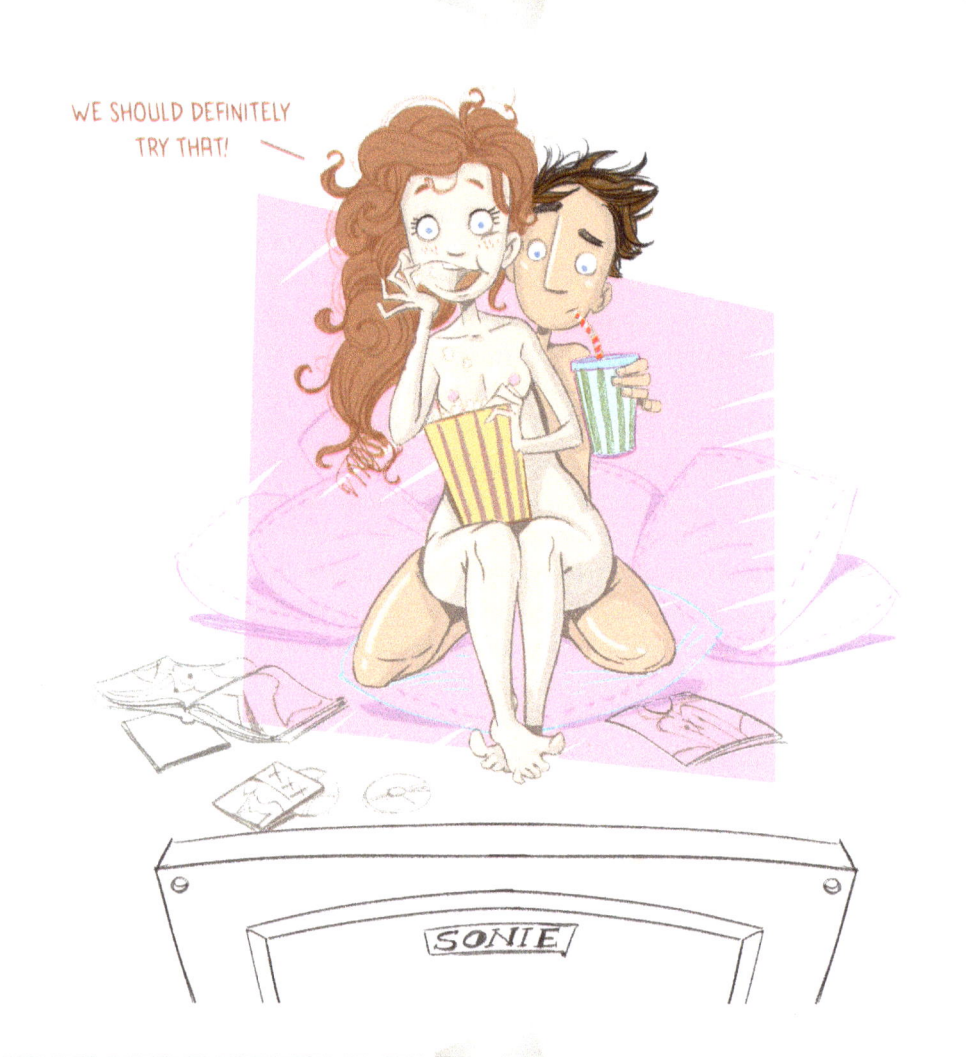

potent panini

easy
20 min

- 6 portobello mushrooms, thinly sliced
- butter, for frying
- 2 panini
- 2 eggs
- 2 cups gruyere cheese, grated
- sprig fresh thyme, chopped
- salt and pepper
- balsamic reduction for drizzling

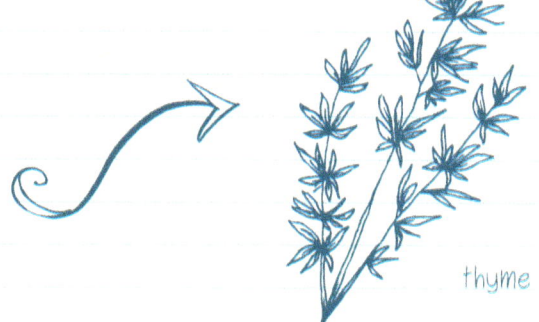
thyme

Fry the mushrooms in butter until crispy. Cut each panini lengthways into three slices. Whisk the eggs and coat each slice in egg. Pan fry the bread in butter until golden. Arrange the bread on a plate, sprinkle with grated cheese and thyme. Top with the mushrooms, season and drizzle with a little balsamic reduction.

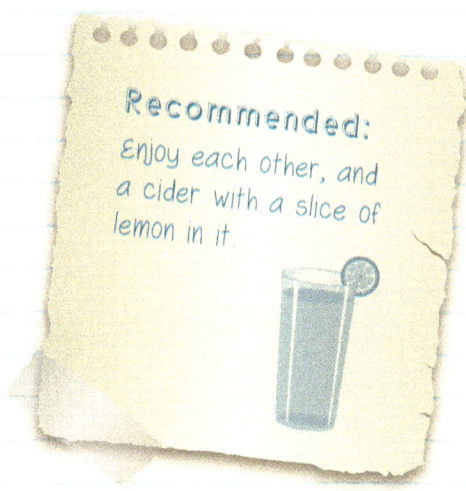

Recommended: Enjoy each other, and a cider with a slice of lemon in it.

The Artist

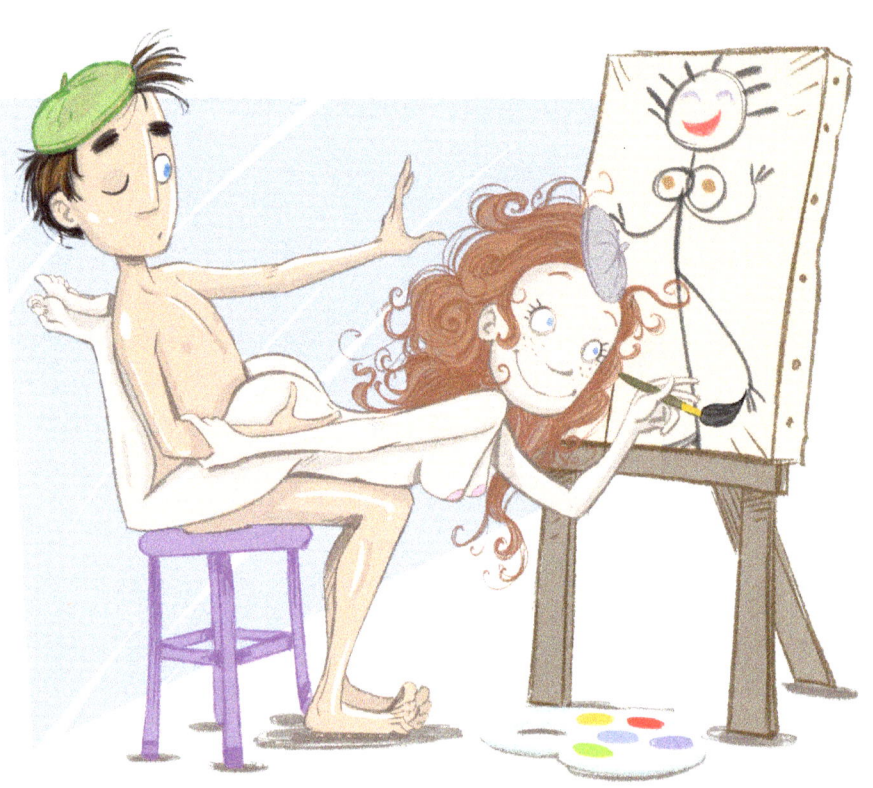

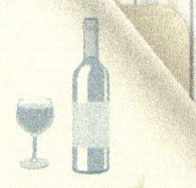

baked camembert 2 die 4

a little effort
30 min

- 300g camembert wheel
- 1 knob unsalted butter, melted
- 3 tbsp sugar
- ¼ cup dried cranberries, roughly chopped
- ¼ cup toasted walnuts, roughly chopped
- sprig fresh rosemary, finely chopped
- sprig fresh thyme, finely chopped
- pinch of salt
- french bread, cut into bite-sized chunks
- 4 rosemary stems, leaves picked off and saved

Using a sharp knife, cut off the top of the Camembert wheel. Place it cut-side up in an ovenproof dish of similar size and height. Combine the melted butter and sugar and stir in the cranberries, nuts, fresh rosemary, thyme and salt. Top the cheese wheel with the cranberry mix. Pop it in the oven at 180°C for 15 minutes or until it is nice and gooey inside. Garnish with rosemary leaves.

Thread the bread onto the rosemary stems and lightly toast them under the grill, just until golden. Dip the bread into the cheese to enjoy.

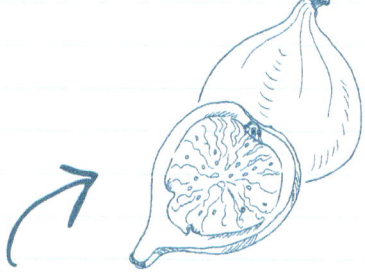

Fresh figs have a voluptuous shape, sweet dark flesh and honey scent that pairs well with this dish. Serve alongside your baked Camembert and feed your lover with this erotic flavour sensation.

THE LOVE BIRDS

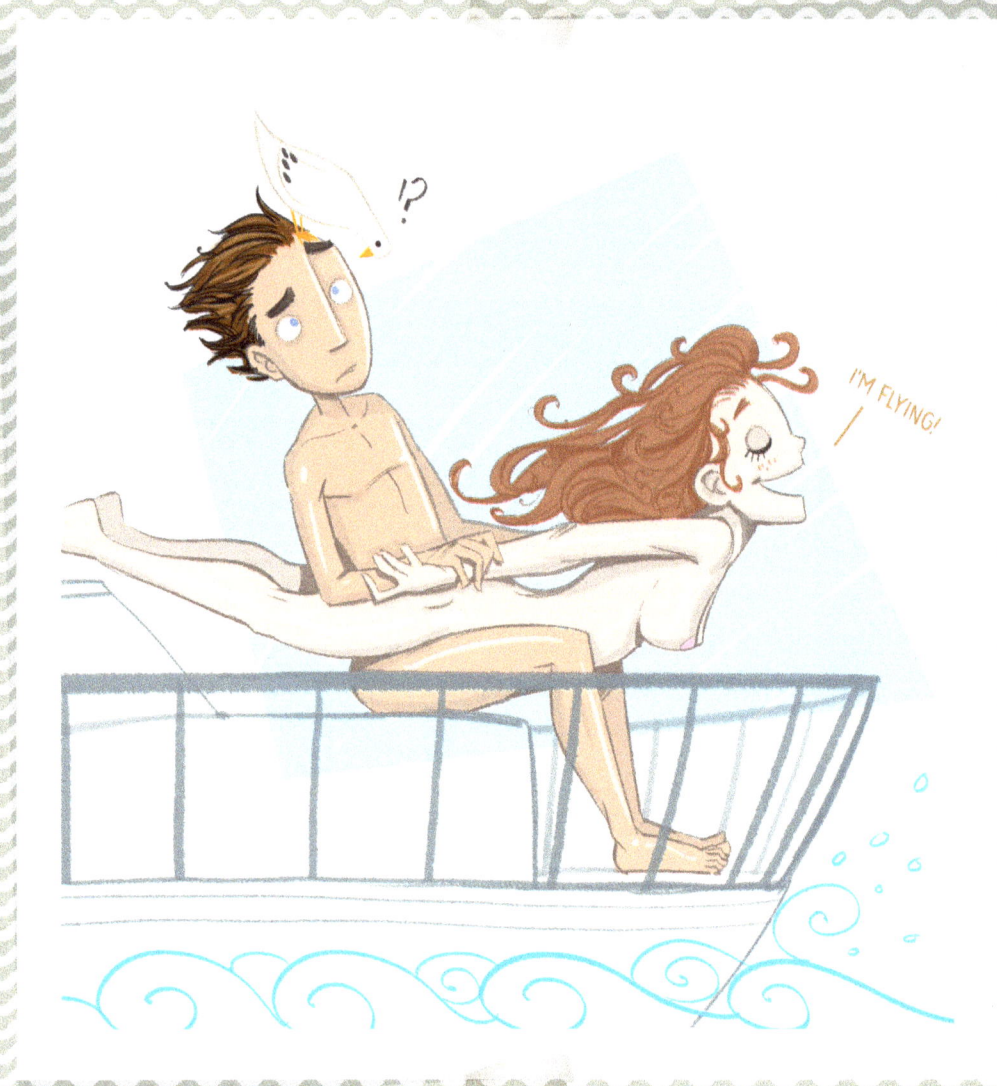

duo terrine

a lot of effort

> 60 min

- ¼ cup full-fat cream cheese
- 1 cup crème fraîche
- 2 tbsp fresh dill, finely chopped
- sprig of coriander, leaves picked and finely chopped
- 1 tbsp horseradish cream
- 2 tsp gelatine
- salt and pepper
- 300g smoked salmon ribbons
- 300g smoked trout ribbons
- 1 cucumber, peeled and sliced into ribbons
- sprig coriander, for garnishing
- savoury biscuits, for serving

In a bowl, mix the cream cheese, crème fraîche, herbs and horseradish. Prepare the gelatine as per instructions on the packet. Stir the gelatine mixture into the cheese mixture and season to taste. Line a rectangular glass dish with cling film so that the plastic overlaps enough to wrap up the terrine. Line the bottom and sides of the dish with overlapping layers of fish, alternating between salmon and trout. Put a layer of overlapping cucumber ribbons over the fish layer. Spoon half the cheese mixture over the layers and even out with a spatula. Repeat the layers and cheese, ending with a layer of fish. Wrap the terrine in the cling film to close it and place a weight on top (e.g. a bag of rice). Put the terrine into the fridge overnight to set. Turn it out, garnish and serve on a wooden platter with your favourite biscuits.

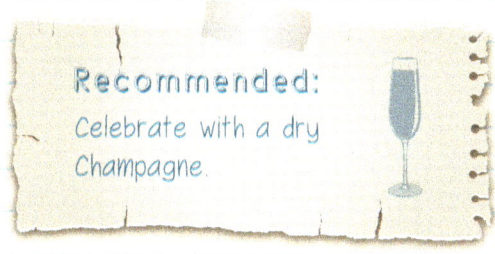

Recommended: Celebrate with a dry Champagne.

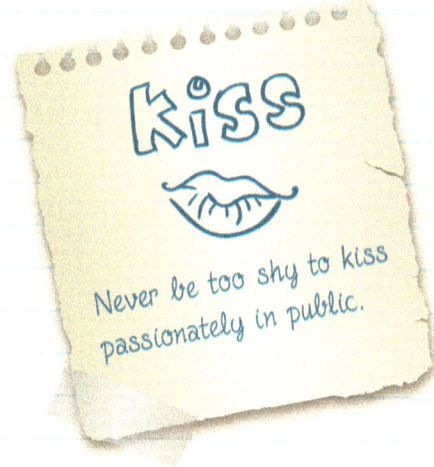

Kiss

Never be too shy to kiss passionately in public.

The Channel Hog

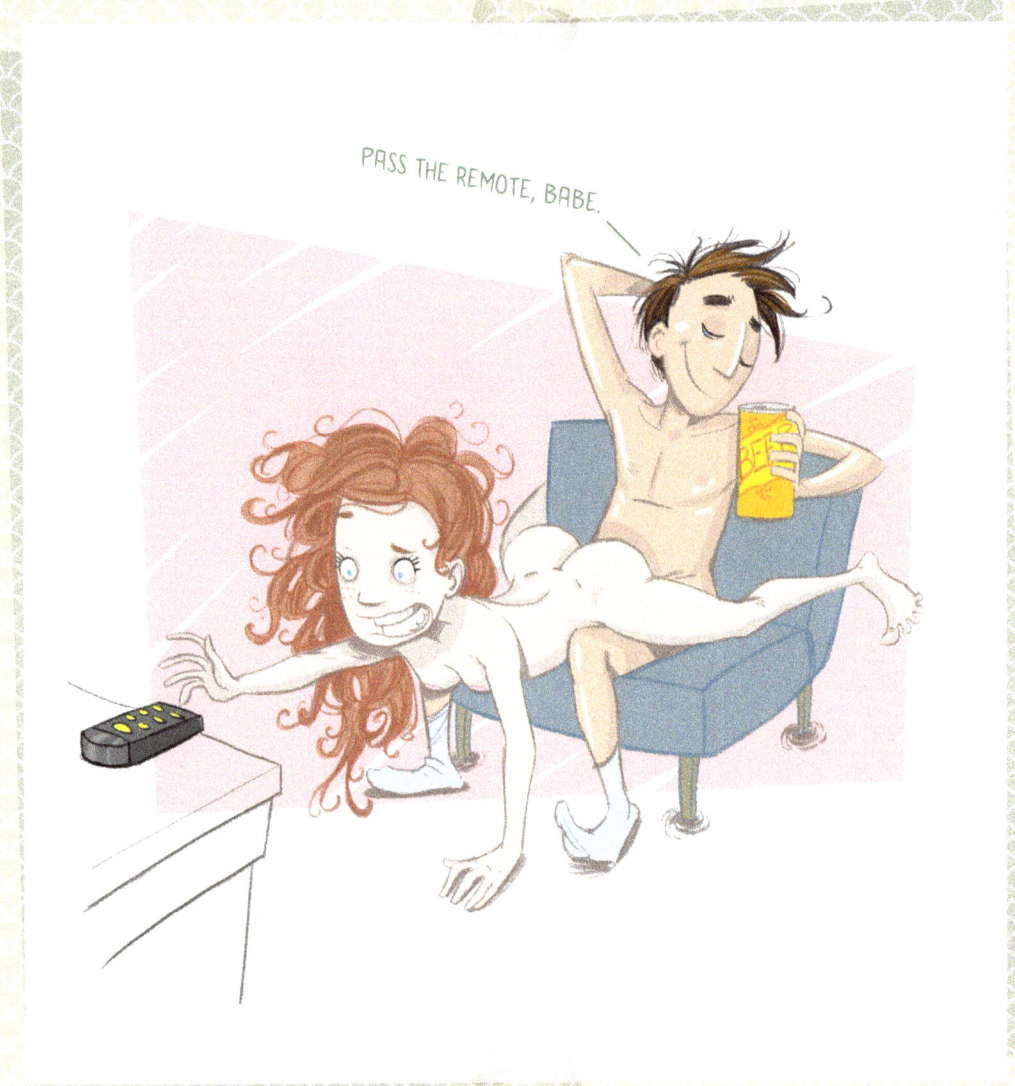

bacon butty

easy
15 min

- 4 rashers streaky bacon
- 2 ripe bananas, cut lengthways
- unsalted butter, at room temperature, for spreading
- 4 slices white bread
- 2 tbsp hp sauce
- dash of tabasco sauce

Reel your partner in with this good, old-fashioned man-bait.

Fry the bacon in its own fat, turning often until nice and crispy. When the bacon is done, transfer it to paper towel and pat gently to drain off the excess fat. Place the bacon on a warming tray to stay warm. Fry the bananas in the bacon fat until golden and soft, turning only once. Butter the bread, layer two slices with the rashes of bacon and drizzle with HP Sauce and a smidgen of tabasco. Close the bacon sandwich and slice into two halves. Repeat with the remaining slices of bread. Serve the bacon butties alongside the slices of banana.

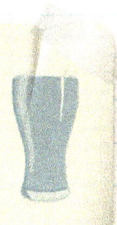

Recommended:
Devour slowly with a craft beer in hand.

THE EXTREME MAKEOVER

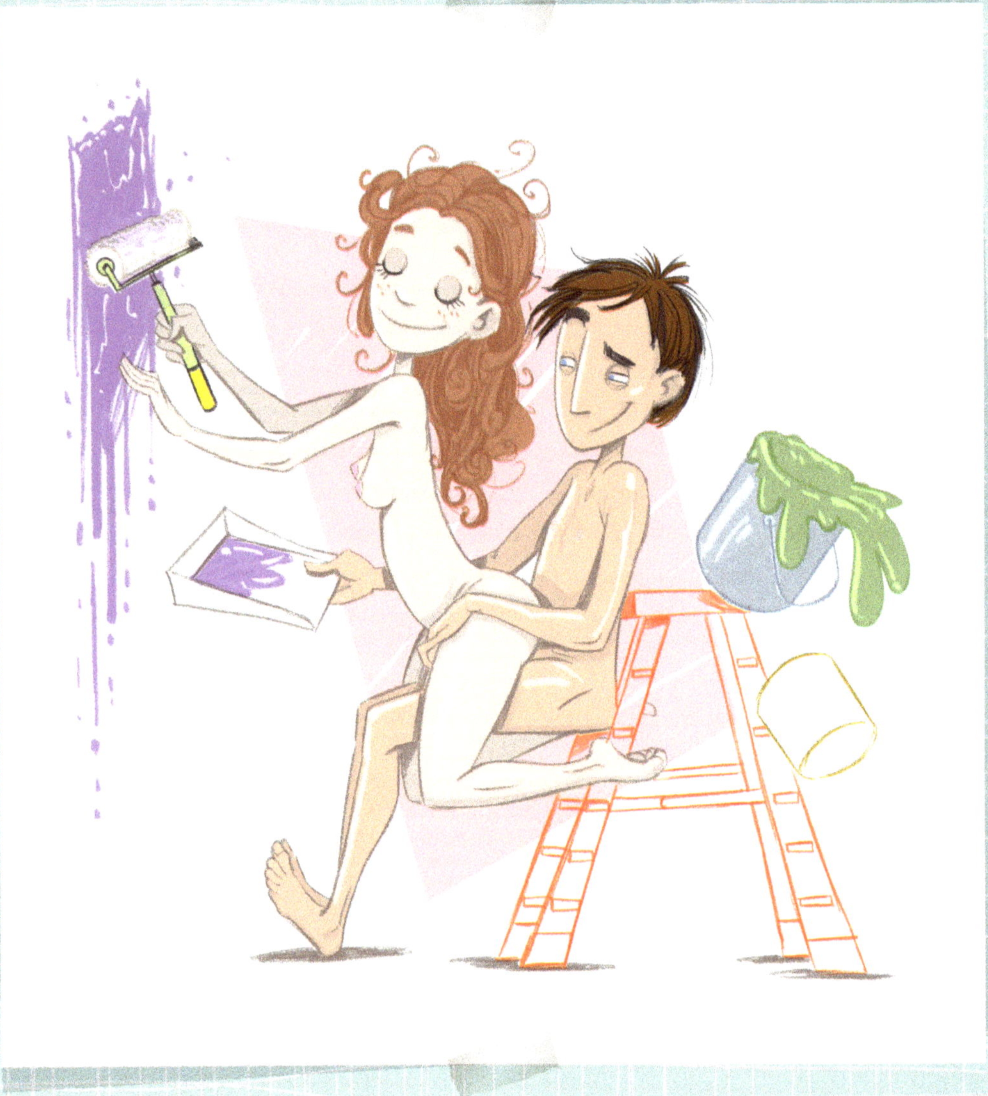

Recommended:
Find a spot on the floor to enjoy your finger foods and serve with a crisp, dry Rosé.

mix-it-up meze

a little effort

45 min

SALAD
- 2 tbsp bulgar wheat
- 1 large ripe tomato, chopped
- handful fresh flat leaf parsley, leaves picked and finely chopped
- handful fresh mint, leaves picked and finely chopped
- ½ red onion, peeled and finely chopped
- 2 tbsp lemon juice
- 2 tbsp good-quality olive oil
- salt and pepper

HALLOUMI SKEWERS
- 4 batons halloumi cheese
- olive oil for drizzling
- ½ tsp paprika
- sprig of fresh lemon thyme

FOR SERVING
- ¼ cup marinated feta
- 4 pita breads, cut into quarters
- handful of seeded savoury biscuits
- ¼ cup stuffed peppadews
- ¼ cup mixed olives
- ¼ cup marinated artichokes
- 4 store-bought dolmades
- ¼ cup store-bought hummus
- 6 slices chorizo sausage

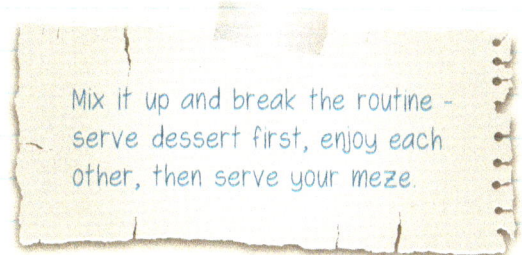

Mix it up and break the routine – serve dessert first, enjoy each other, then serve your meze.

For the salad, place the bulgar wheat in a small bowl and cover with boiling water. Cover with a plate and allow to steam for 20 minutes. When it has absorbed all the water, fluff it up with a fork. Combine the tomato, parsley, mint and onion in a bowl. Toss with the bulgar wheat, add the lemon juice and olive oil and season. Toss again to coat the ingredients in the dressing.

For the halloumi skewers, thread the halloumi onto 4 skewers that have been soaked in water. Drizzle with olive oil and sprinkle over the paprika and thyme, coating all sides. Bring a griddle pan to a medium heat, and grill the cheese giving the batons nice grill marks and warming them through.

Prepare a large wooden board with the salad, cheese, bread and biscuits, peppadews, olives, artichokes, dolmades, hummus and sausage.

The Lotus Surprise

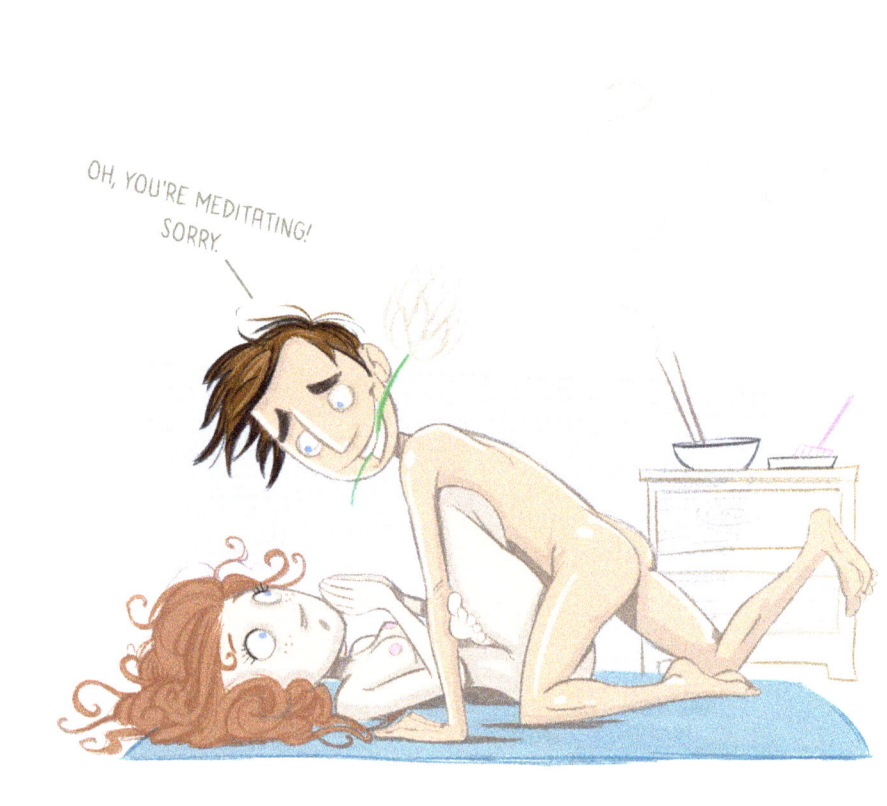

wanton noodles

easy
20 min

- 4 courgettes, sliced julienne
- 2 baby marrows, sliced julienne
- quick-cook chinese noodles
- knob of butter
- thai spice
- black pepper
- ½ sweet red pepper, sliced julienne
- handful fresh coriander leaves
- 2 tbsp cream cheese

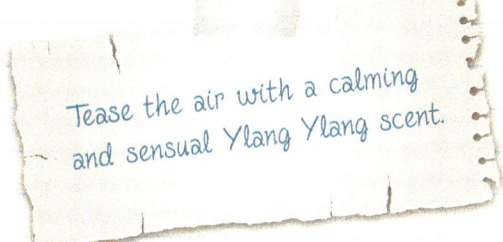

Tease the air with a calming and sensual Ylang Ylang scent.

Cook the courgettes and marrows for a minute in a microwave oven. Boil the noodles as per instructions on the packet and drain. Melt the butter with the spice and pepper in a pan, and add the veggies. Fry for a minute and add the noodles. Stir-fry veggies and noodles for an additional 2 minutes, then add the coriander leaves. Spoon on some cream cheese and enjoy.

Recommended:
Delicious served with lemonade poured over crushed ice and a dash of grenadine. Garnish with a slice of orange, a swizzle stick and two straws.

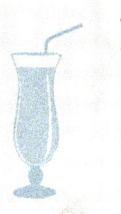

The Hole In One

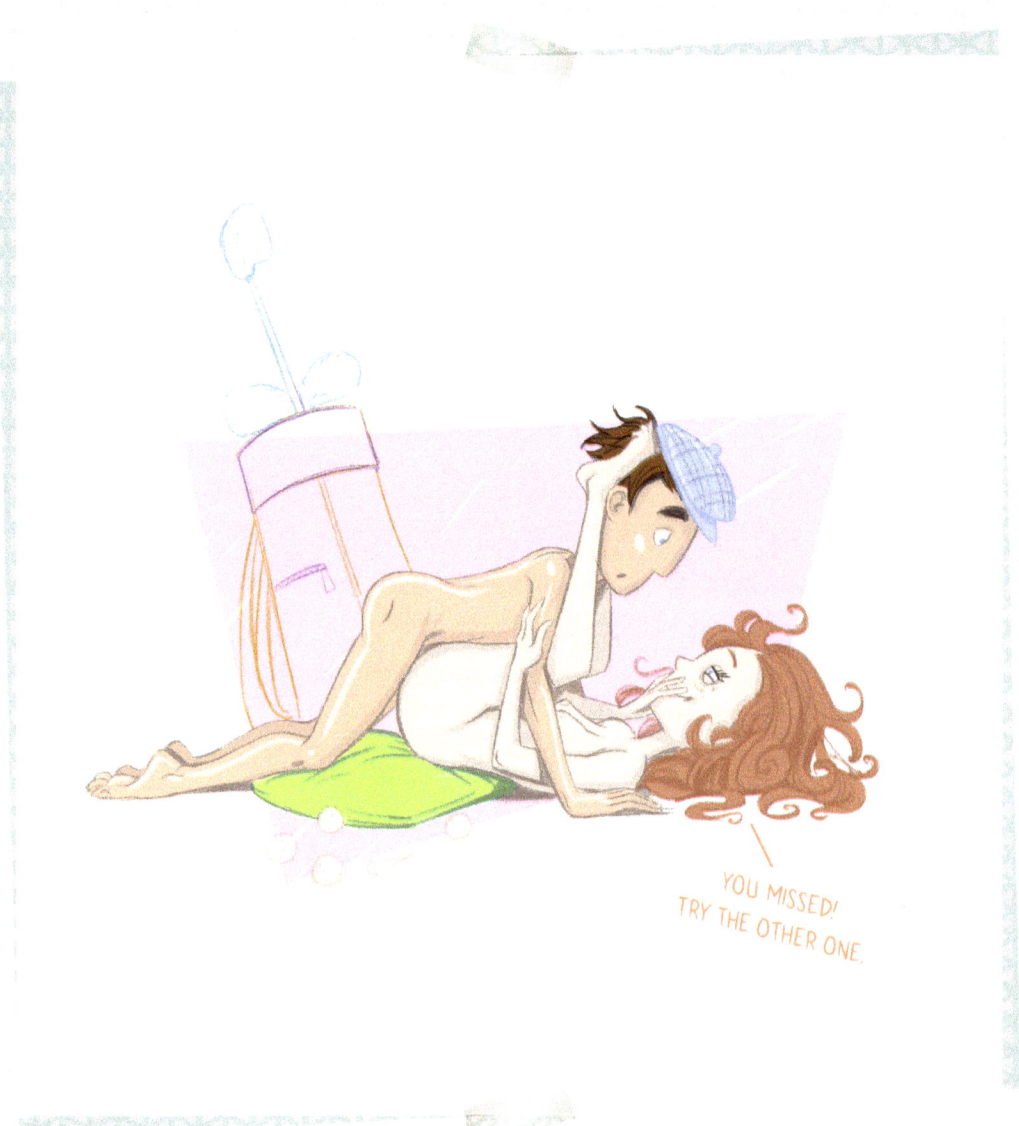

devilish hearts

easy

25 min

- 1½ cup preserved artichoke hearts, drained
- 2 tbsp good-quality mayonnaise
- ½ cup parmesan cheese, grated
- salt and pepper
- ciabatta, sliced

Arrange the artichoke hearts in a shallow, ovenproof dish. Spoon the mayonnaise on top and mix. Layer with cheese and season to taste. Pop into the oven for 15 minutes at 180°C and then grill for an additional 3 minutes until golden. Serve warm on toasted ciabatta.

Build anticipation by exchanging flirty texts before you see each other.

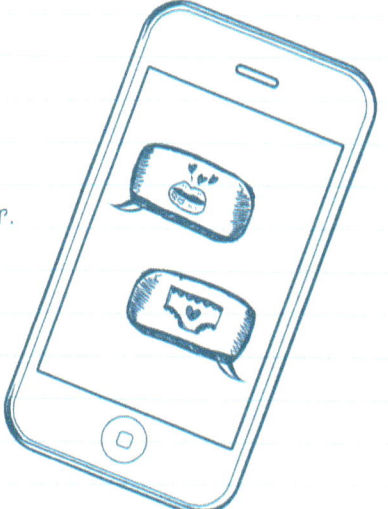

Recommended:
If you are in the mood for wine, crack open an unwooded Chardonnay.

THE SECRET

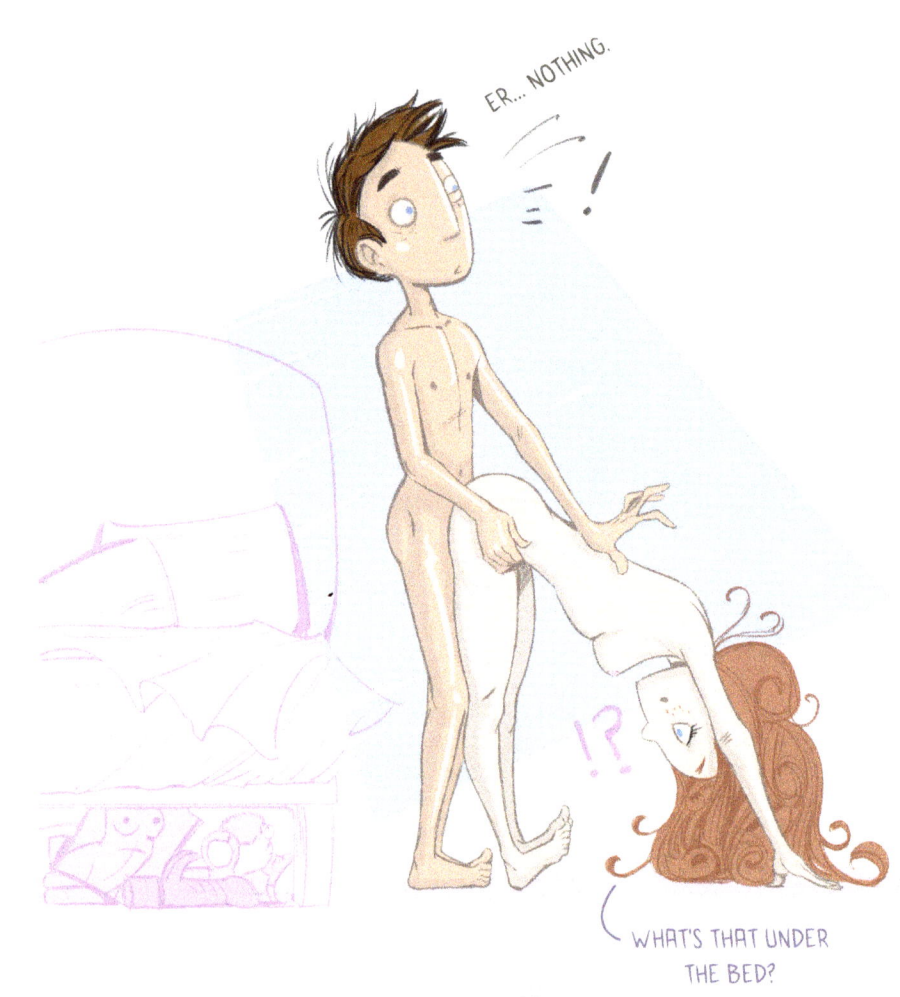

macho gazpacho

easy
> 60 min

- 1 red onion, peeled and chopped
- 2 sticks celery, chopped
- 1 red pepper, seeds removed and chopped
- 1 medium cucumber, chopped
- 2 cups ripe italian tomatoes, chopped
- 2 tsp tabasco sauce
- 2 cloves of garlic, crushed
- 2 cups tomato juice
- ¼ cup white wine vinegar
- ¼ cup good quality olive oil
- 2 tsp course salt
- 2 twists ground black pepper
- 2 slices crisp flat bread

Blitz the onion, celery, red pepper, cucumber and tomato in a food processor. Don't over-do it, it must end up a coarse mixture. Pour the mixture into a large bowl and stir in the remaining ingredients. Put the soup into the fridge for at least two hours and serve in small bowls or mugs with the bread.

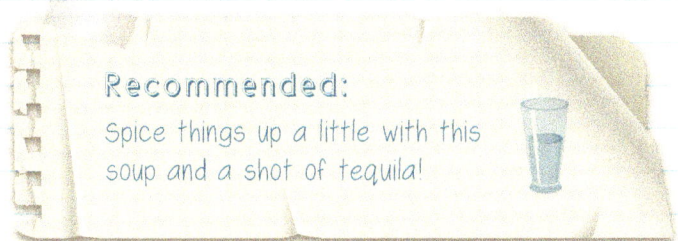

Recommended:
Spice things up a little with this soup and a shot of tequila!

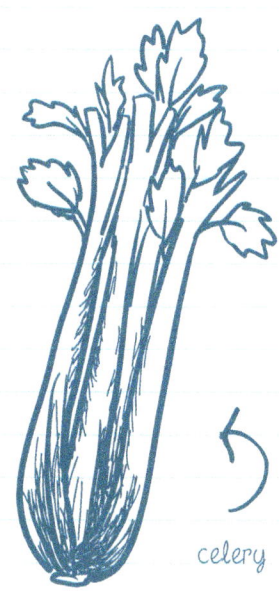

celery

The Sneaky Bastard

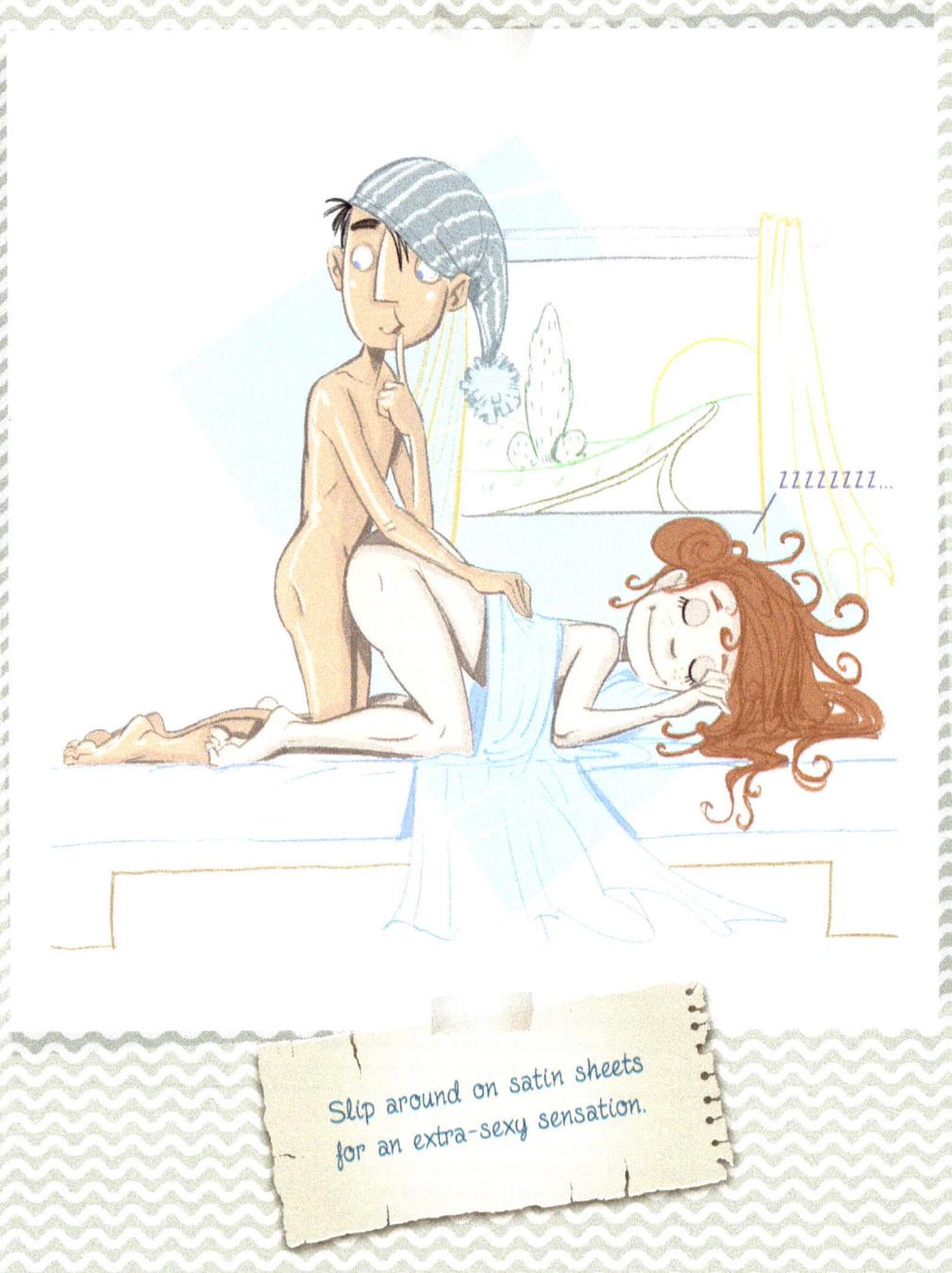

Slip around on satin sheets for an extra-sexy sensation.

quickie turkey sandwich

easy
15 min

- 4 slices cooked turkey breast, diced
- handful of baby tomatoes, quartered
- 1 tbsp mayonnaise
- handful fresh rocket, coarsely chopped
- sprig fresh thyme, leaves picked from the stem
- salt and pepper
- 2 slices health bread
- cucumber, sliced into ribbons
- sprig fresh basil

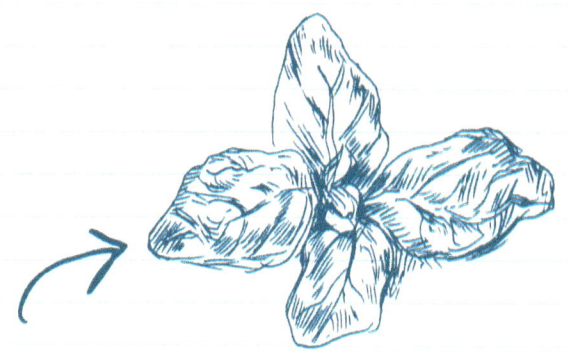

basil

In a bowl, mix the turkey, tomatoes, mayonnaise, rocket and thyme. Season to taste. Lightly toast the bread, top with cucumber ribbons and give it a thick layer of the turkey topping. Garnish with basil.

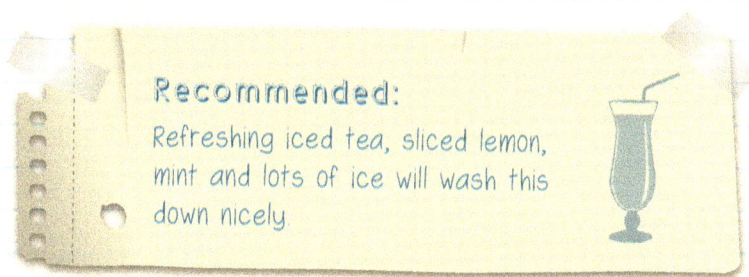

Recommended:
Refreshing iced tea, sliced lemon, mint and lots of ice will wash this down nicely.

The Sun Goddess

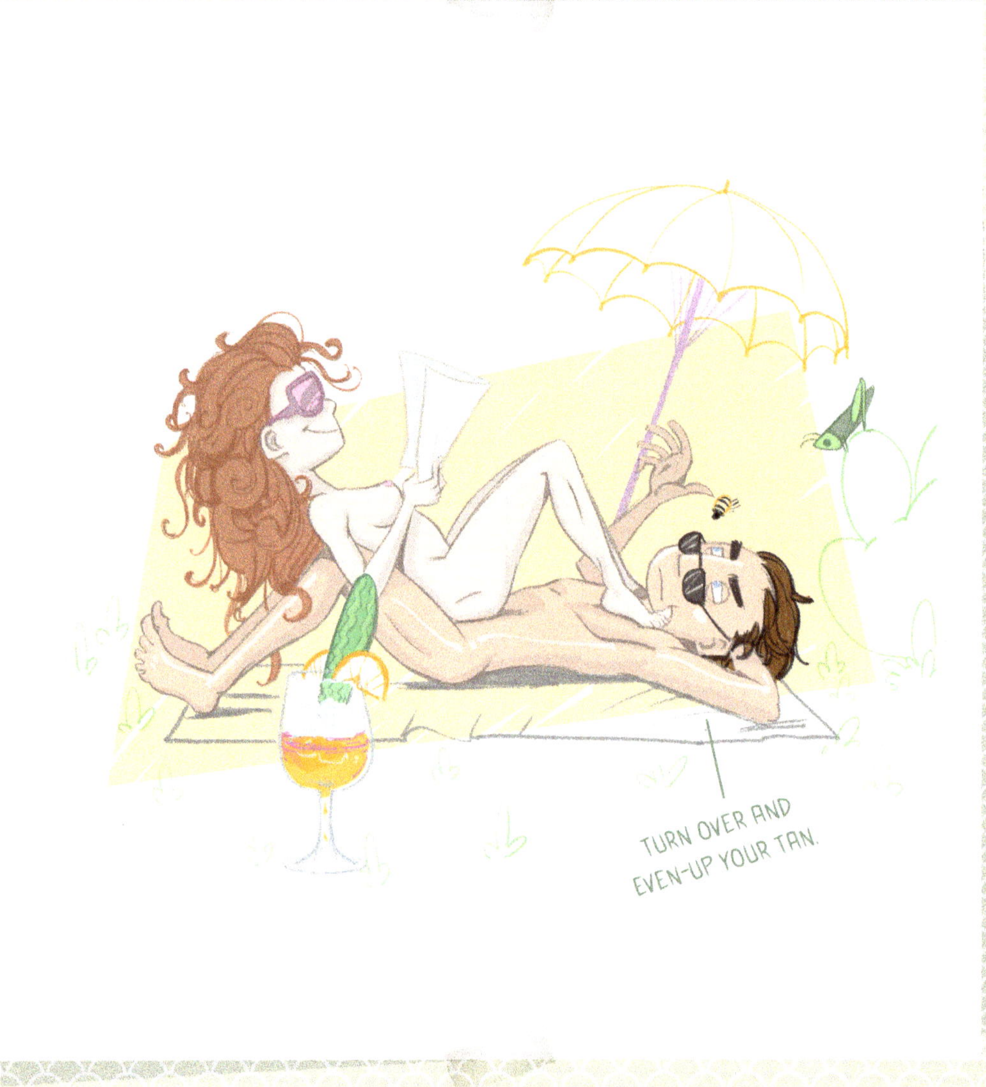

TURN OVER AND EVEN-UP YOUR TAN.

Salmon is a great choice with which to peak your sex-hormone production.

moist and fiery salmon

a little effort
> 60 min

- 3 tbsp soy sauce
- 3 tbsp medium-cream sherry
- 4 salmon fillets, skinned and deboned
- 1 cucumber, peeled and seeds removed
- 1 red chilli, finely chopped
- 2 tsp sugar
- 4 tbsp rice vinegar
- thumb fresh ginger, peeled and grated
- salt and pepper
- handful fresh coriander leaves, coarsely chopped
- 2 large potatoes, baked in their jackets and seasoned
- knob of butter for the potato
- 1 cup of mixed vegetables, steamed

Combine the soy and sherry in a small jug. Place the fillets in a shallow bowl and pour over the soy and sherry mixture to coat each piece. Cover the bowl and put it in the fridge to marinate for 2 hours. Slice the cucumber and place it in a bowl with the chilli, sugar, vinegar, ginger and seasoning. Remove the salmon from the fridge and fry it in a heavy-based pan ensuring it is still moist on the inside. Plate the salmon and pour the remaining marinade over it. Garnish with the coriander. Serve on a hot day with the jacket potato and vegetables.

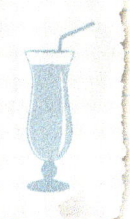

Recommended:
Make a thirst quenching cocktail with 45ml Pimm's, topped up with lemonade and served over crushed ice. A stick of cucumber and sliced orange in the glass will add some colour.

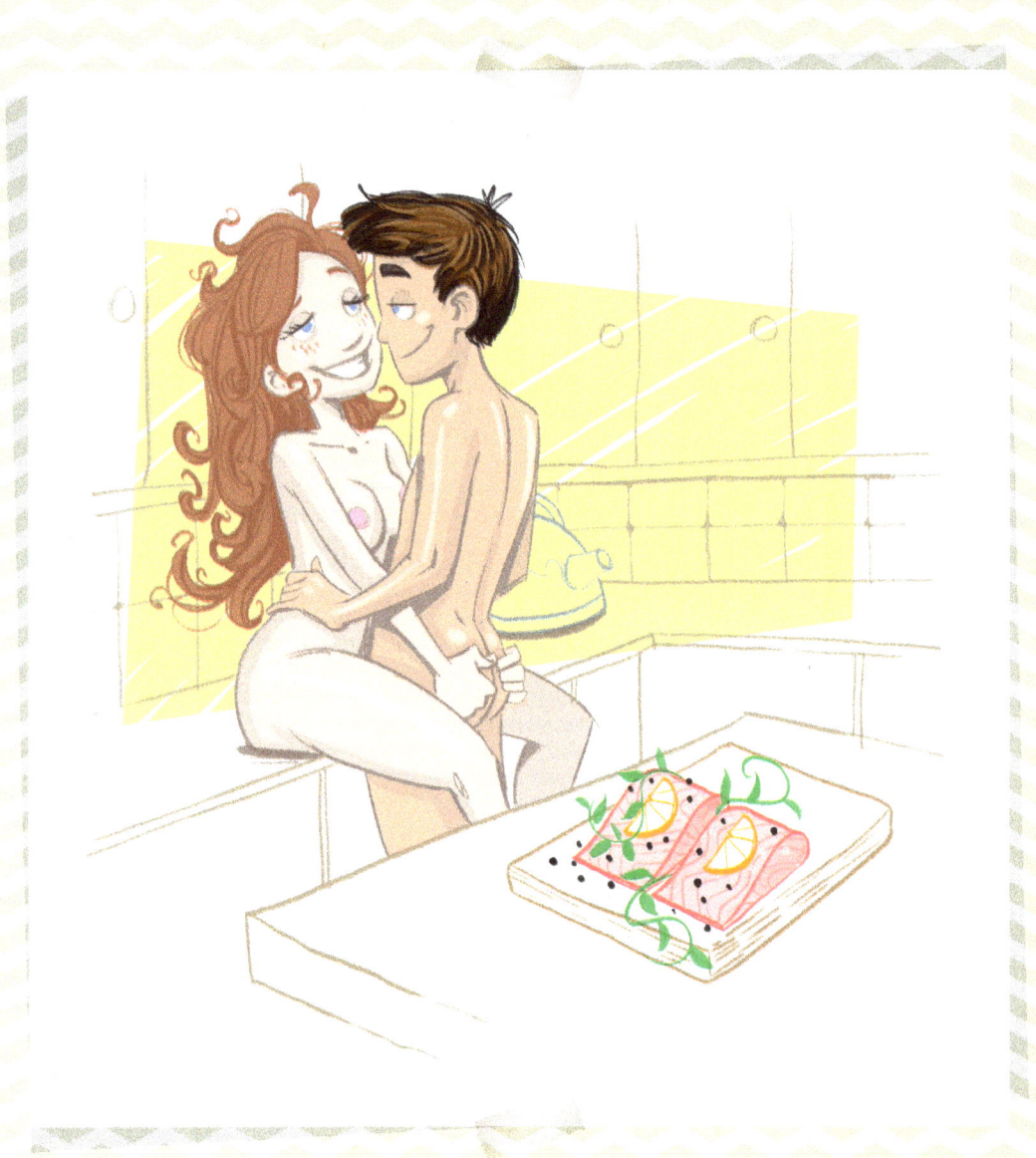

Marinating time is perfect hanky-panky time!

The Dragon Tamer

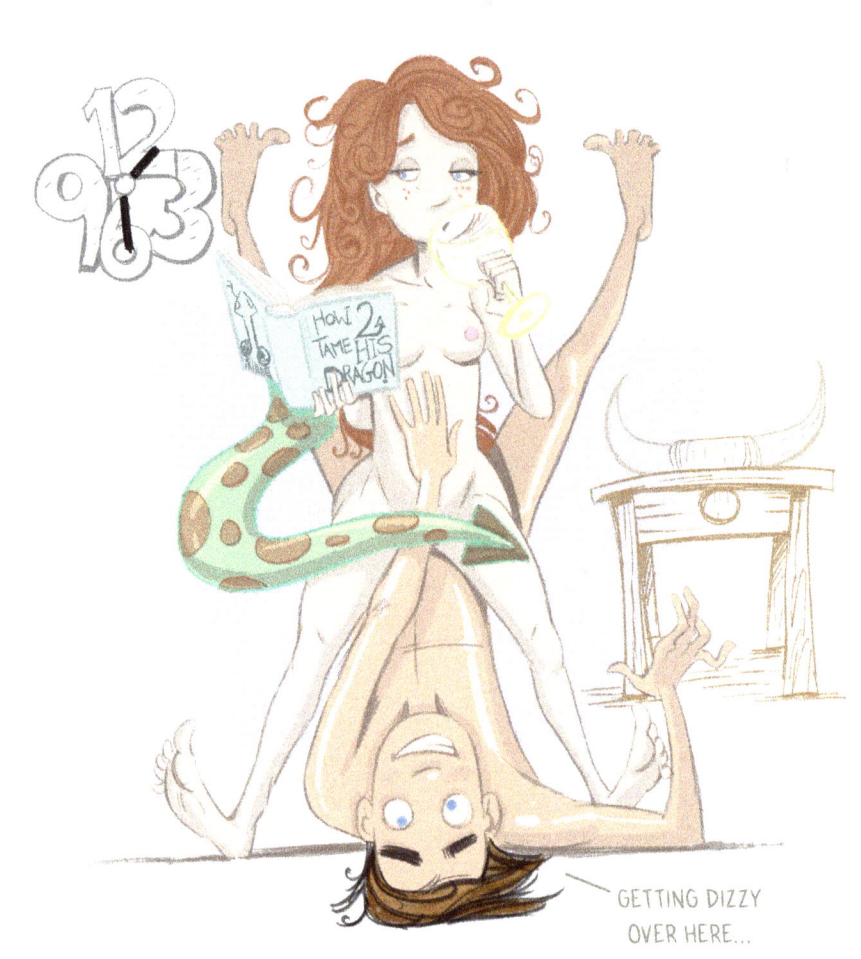

silky tomato soup

a little effort

\> 60 min

- olive oil, for drizzling
- 3 cups ripe italian tomatoes
- salt and pepper
- 1 onion, peeled and chopped
- 1 tsp garlic, crushed
- knob of butter
- 1½ cups chicken stock
- 2 sprigs fresh thyme, leaves picked from the stem
- handful fresh basil, chopped
- ½ cup double-thick cream
- ciabatta, sliced
- 6 slices mozzarella cheese
- 1 tsp dried italian herbs

Drizzle oil over the tomatoes, season and pop in the oven at 180°C until soft. Fry the onions and garlic in butter until translucent. Allow the tomatoes to cool, peel off the skins and put them in a large pot. Add the stock, fresh herbs and a little seasoning and bring to a simmer for about 10 minutes. Use a hand blender to blitz the mixture into a smooth soup. Add the cream and stir well. Cover the ciabatta slices with the mozzarella and sprinkle over some dried herbs. Grill the slices until the cheese has melted, then serve with the soup.

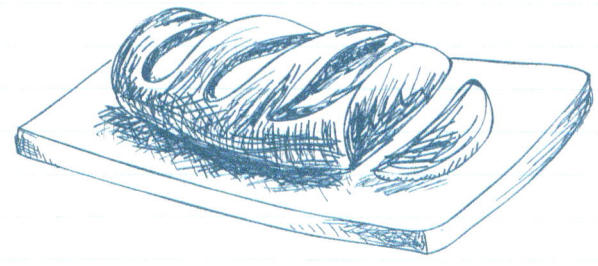

Recommended:
Tease the taste buds with a Noble Late Harvest.

The Free Ride

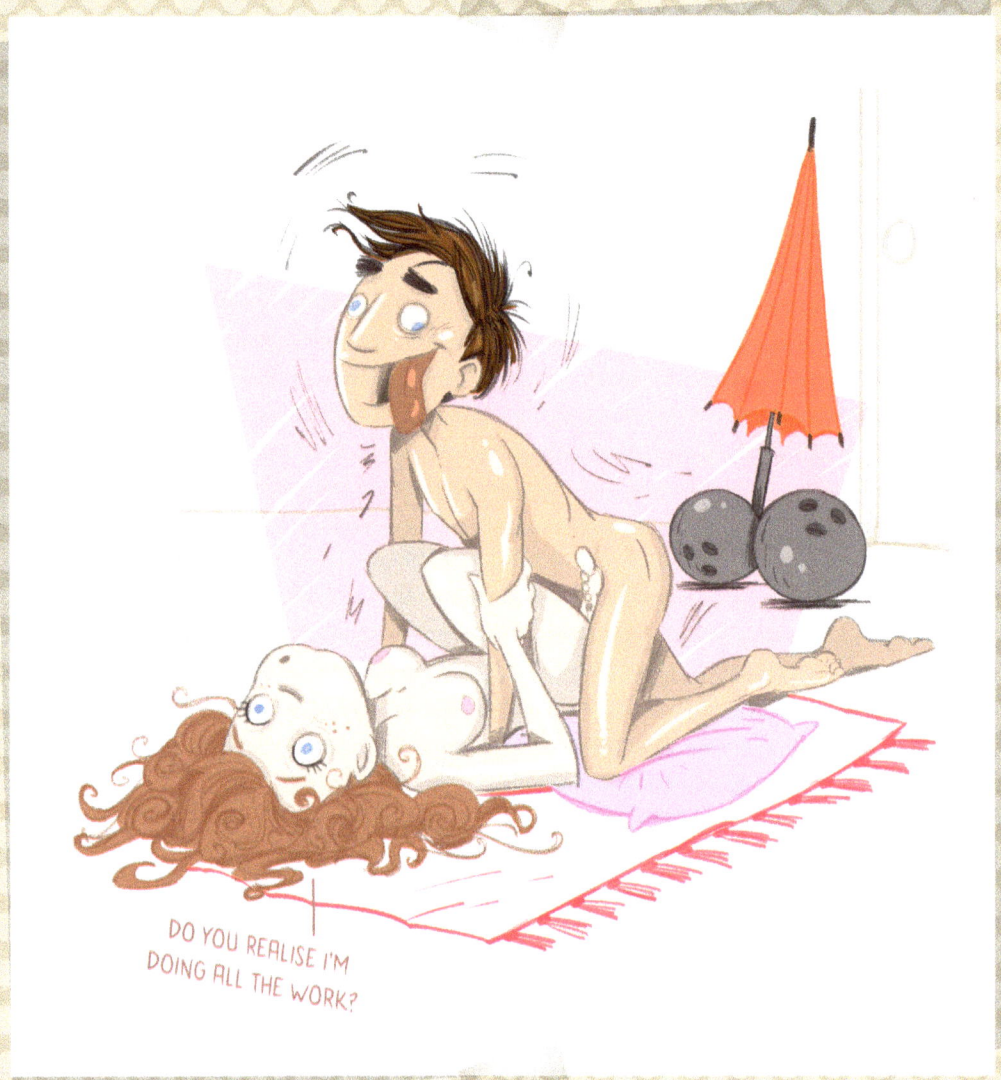

tantalising tagliolini

easy
25 min

- 1 avocado pear, mashed
- 1 tbsp creamy mayonnaise
- handful rocket, roughly chopped
- handful basil, torn into strips
- salt and pepper
- 4 rashers streaky bacon
- 5 rosa tomatoes, halved
- good-quality olive oil
- 1 packet of fresh tagliolini pasta
- ¼ cup pine nuts, toasted
- basil leaves, for garnishing

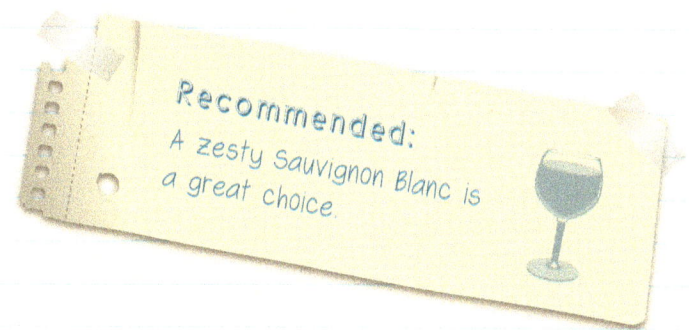

Recommended:
A zesty Sauvignon Blanc is a great choice.

Mix the avocado, mayonnaise and herbs into a paste. Season to taste. Grill the bacon until crispy and then cut it into small pieces. Drizzle the tomatoes with olive oil and grill until soft. Cook the pasta al dente, drain and place in a serving bowl. Toss the pasta with a dash of olive oil and the pine nuts. Top with the avocado mix and bacon pieces. Decorate with the tomatoes and basil.

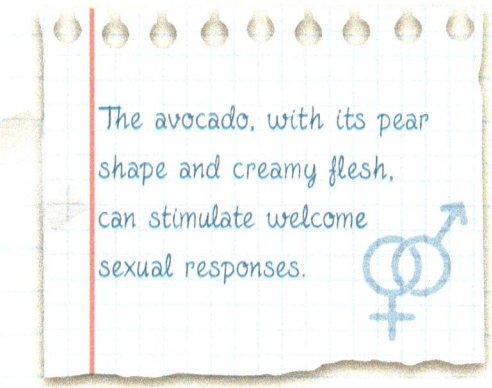

The avocado, with its pear shape and creamy flesh, can stimulate welcome sexual responses.

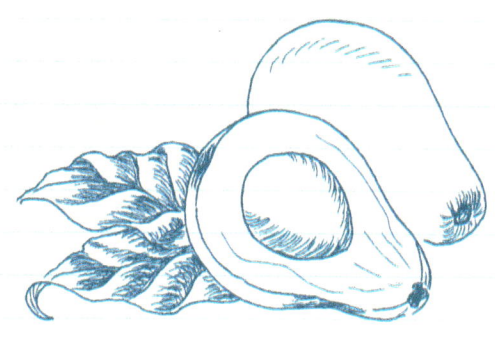

The Hard Yards

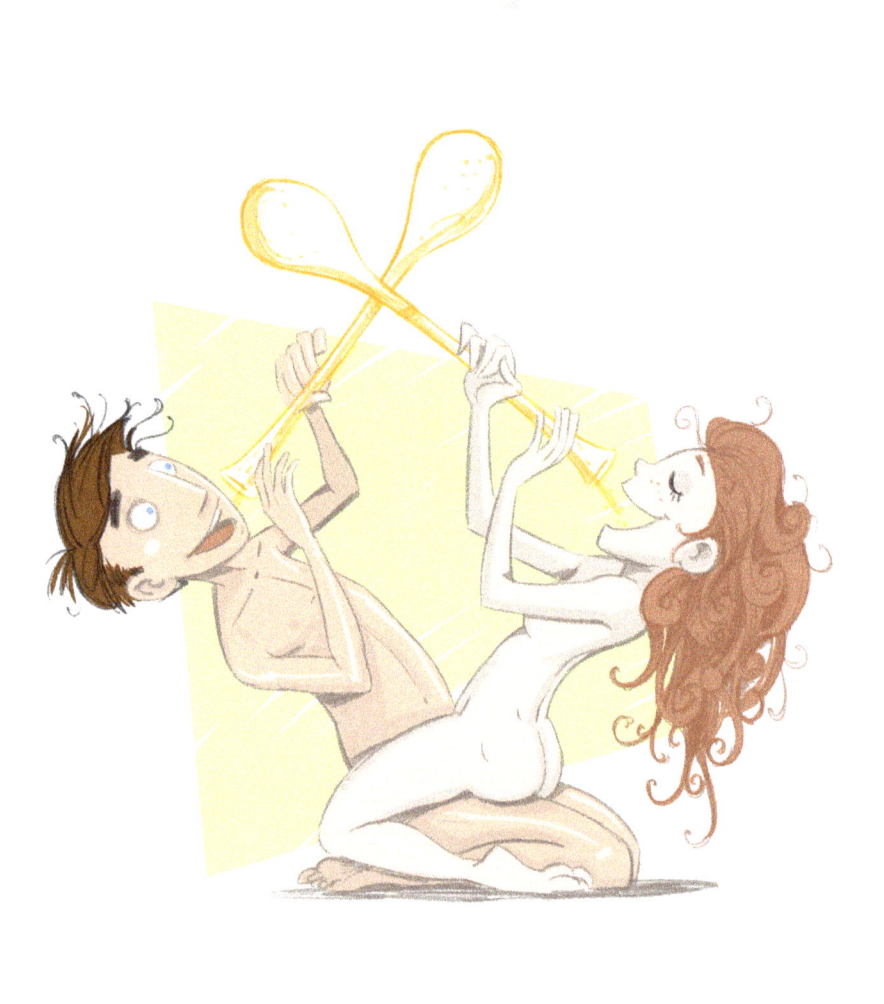

forking fantastic toasties

easy

15 min

- 4 slices ciabatta
- 1 cup double-thick cream
- ½ cup mature cheddar cheese, grated
- ¼ cup gruyere cheese, grated
- 1 tsp hot english mustard
- 2 egg yolks
- salt and pepper
- 1 tbsp worcester sauce
- handful fresh baby rocket

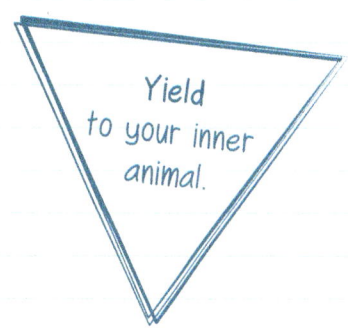

Yield to your inner animal.

Lightly toast the bread. Mix the cream, cheese, mustard and eggs in a large bowl. Top the toasted bread with the mixture and pop the slices under the grill until they are crispy and golden. Cut a grid pattern into the cheesy top, drizzle with Worcester sauce and season. Serve hot, garnished with a few rocket leaves.

Recommended:
Enjoy with a yard of your favourite ale.

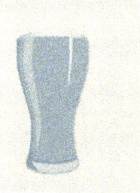

Notes

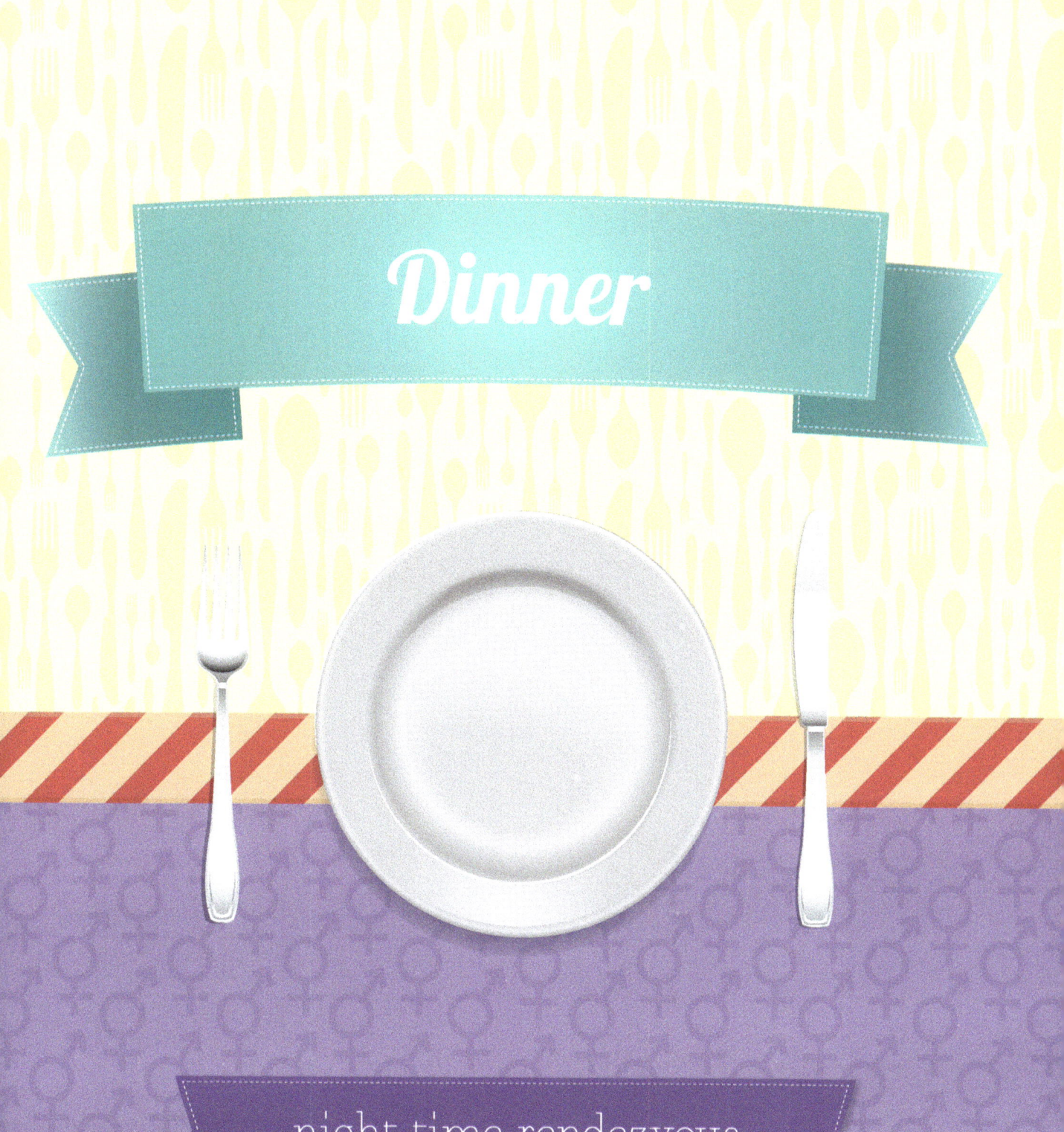

THE DUET

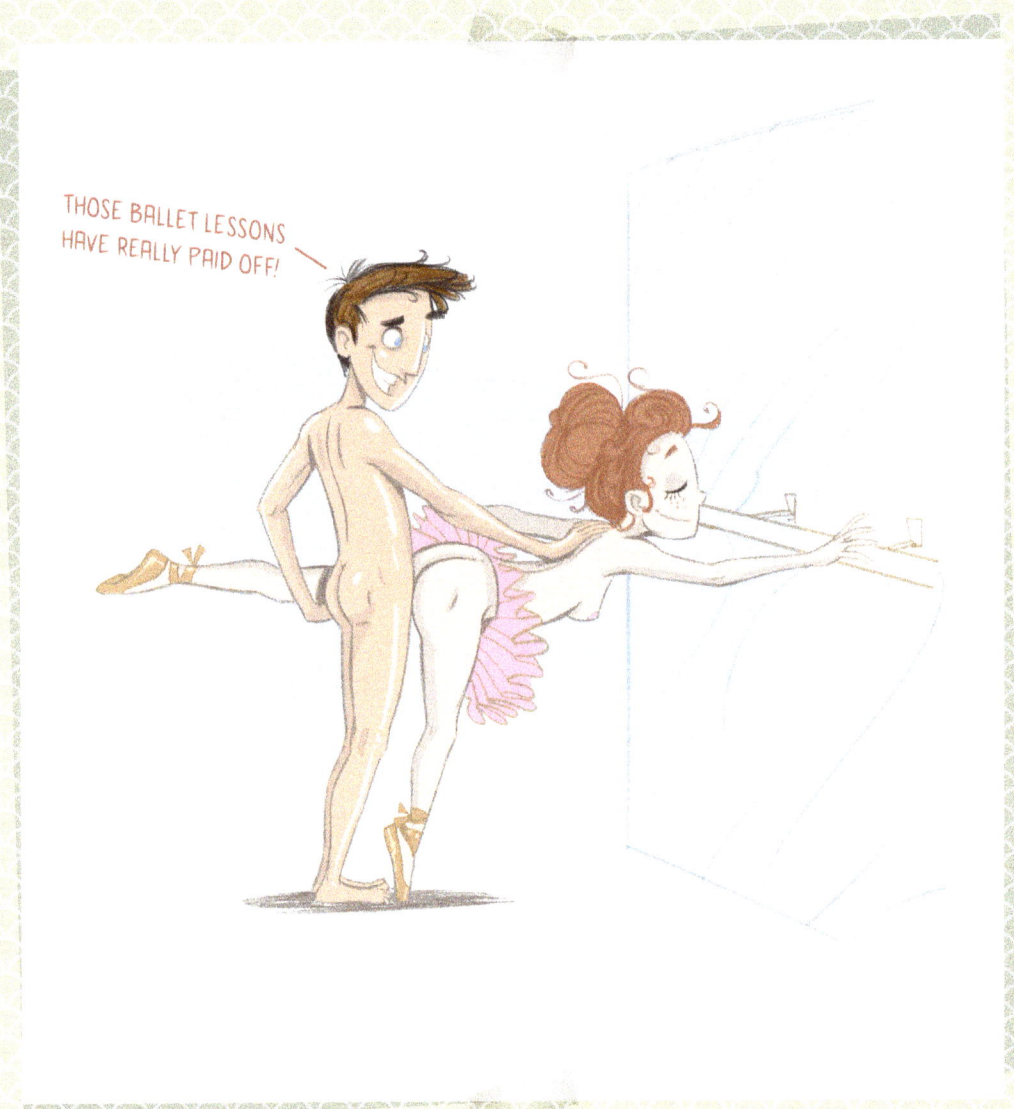

fish with rösti

a little effort
30 min

- 2 potatoes, peeled and grated
- olive oil, for drizzling
- 2 salmon fillets
- fish rub
- salt and pepper
- 2 tbsp japanese mayonnaise
- 1 tsp caviar
- 1 tsp fresh dill, finely chopped

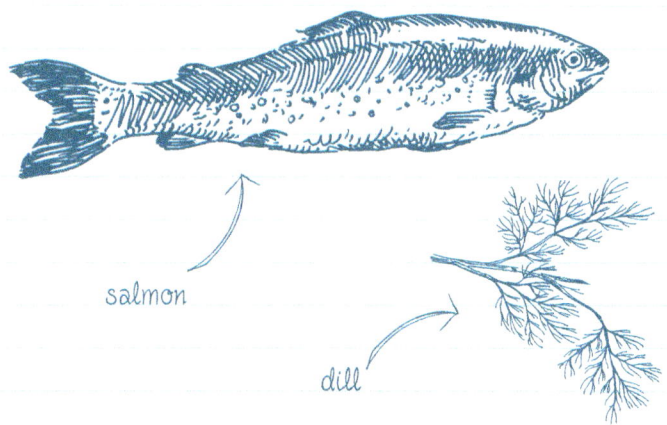

salmon

dill

Squeeze the excess water from the potatoes and form them into two patties. Place them on a greased baking tray, drizzle with olive oil and pop in the oven for 15 minutes on 150°C. Grill for an additional 5 minutes until golden. Massage the fish lovingly with the rub and pan-fry for 2 minutes on each side. Place the röstis on a plate, season and top with the salmon fillets. Garnish with a dollop of mayonnaise and the caviar. Sprinkle with dill.

Recommended:
Pop open some pink Champagne to jazz it up a bit.

The Cheerleader

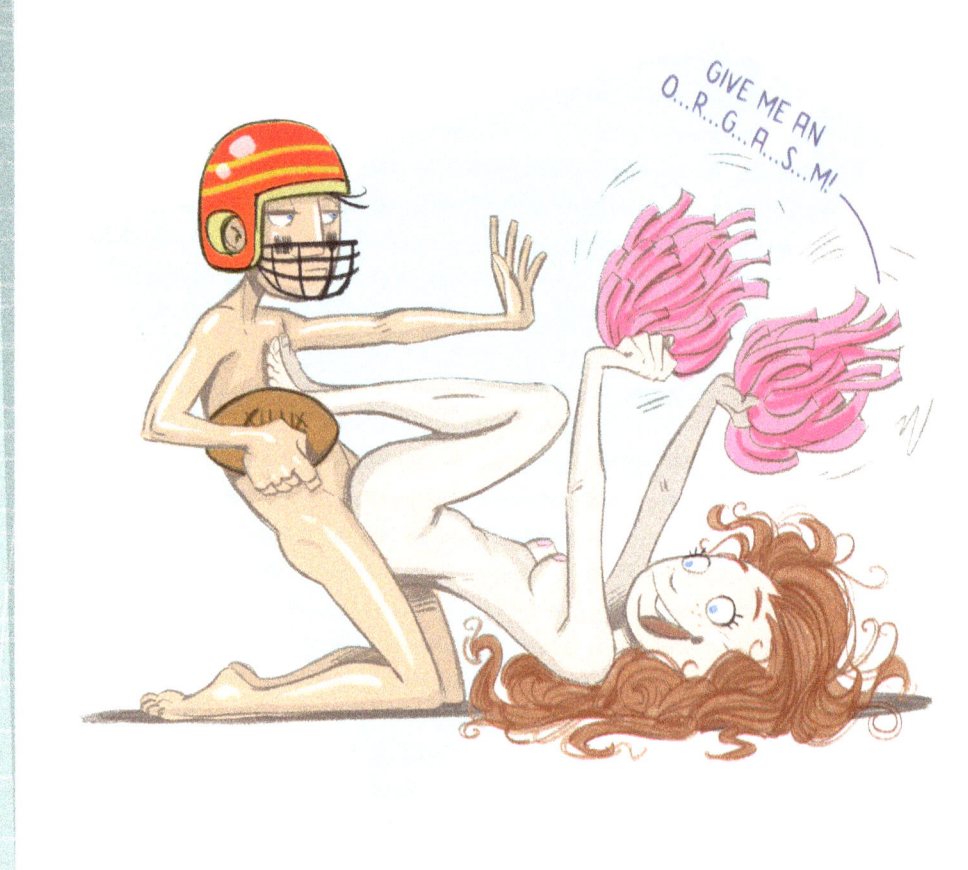

burger deluxe

a little effort

\> 60 min

- 10 crackers, crushed in a plastic bag
- 4 sprigs fresh italian parsley
- 4 sprigs fresh thyme
- 1 green pepper, deseeded and finely chopped
- 3 tsp dijon mustard
- 400g lean beef mince
- 1 egg
- salt and pepper
- 1 tbsp olive oil
- 1 red onion, peeled and sliced
- 2 large slices cheddar cheese
- 2 large burger buns, cut in half
- 2 tbsp creamy mayonnaise
- 2 slices tomato
- ½ head of cos lettuce, shredded

To make the patties, place crackers in a large bowl with the herbs, green pepper, mustard and mince. Add the egg and season. Mix the ingredients by hand until well blended and then divide into 6-8 rounded patties. Pat down the patties with the palm of your hand, drizzle with a little olive oil, cover and put in the fridge for 30 minutes.

In the meantime, sauté your onions in a little olive oil until golden and set aside.

Heat a griddle pan, and fry the patties on a medium heat until cooked through, turning once.

Place the patties, onion and then sliced cheese on the bottom half of the buns and pop under the grill for a few minutes until the cheese has just melted and buns are lightly toasted. Put the top half in at the same time for light toasting. Remove and allow to cool slightly. Spread mayonnaise on the top half and top with tomato and lettuce. Season and serve with a bucket of French fries and your favourite sauce.

> **Recommended:**
> After the game, treat yourselves to a burger, fries and an ice-cold beer.

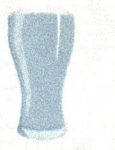

THE WRESTLER

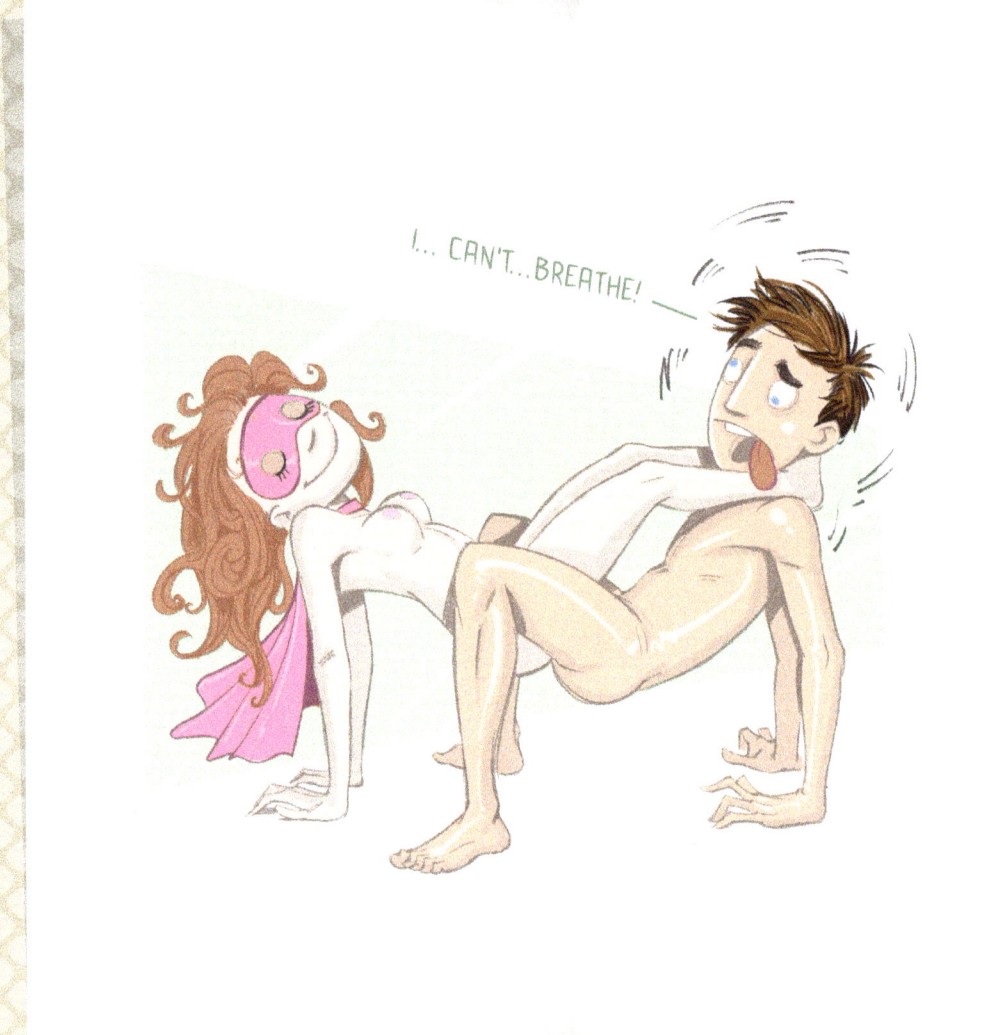

fancy-pants fillet

easy
> 60 min

- 1 can coca-cola
- ½ cup balsamic vinegar
- ¼ cup honey
- 2 sprigs fresh rosemary, leaves picked
- fillet of beef, cut into medallions
- olive oil, for frying
- salt and pepper

SAUCE
- ½ cup milk
- ½ cup cream
- ½ cup creamy gorgonzola or blue cheese
- ½ cup cheddar cheese, grated
- cornflour, if needed

Blitz the coca-cola, vinegar, honey and rosemary together in a food processor. Marinate the fillet in the mixture for 2 hours. Heat a griddle pan and add a glug of olive oil. Season and then cook the fillet to taste. Top with the cheesy sauce and serve.

To make the cheesy sauce, bring the milk and cream to the boil. Add the cheese and allow to melt. Turn down the heat and thicken with cornflour if needed.

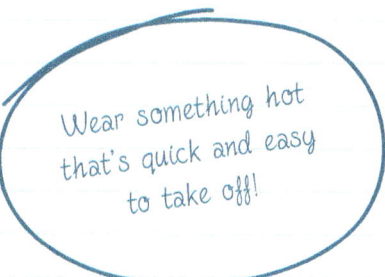

Wear something hot that's quick and easy to take off!

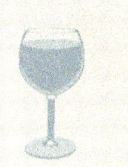

Recommended:
Great served with polenta, steamed vegetables and a generous glass of Merlot.

The Tango

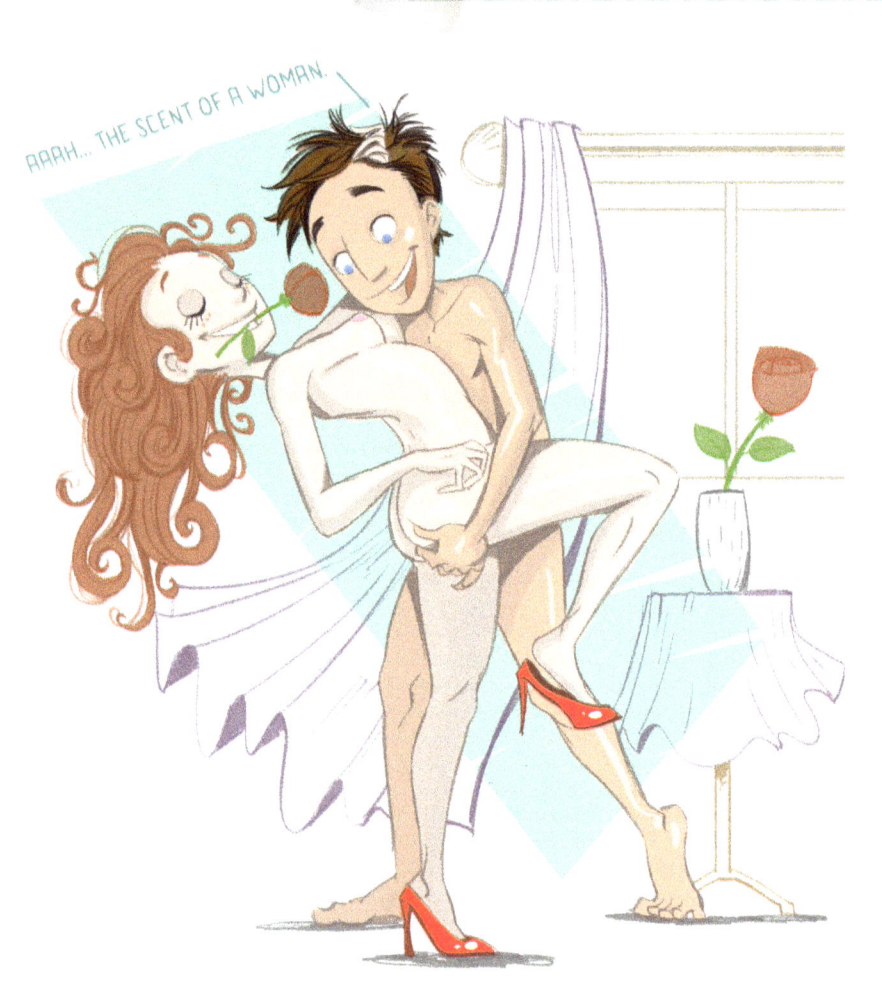

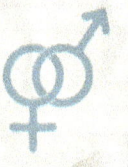

Chilli can get your blood pumping but watch where you put your hands!

drop-your-panties gnocchi

a little effort

40 min

- 1 garlic clove, peeled and sliced
- handful capers, drained and chopped
- 2 handfuls calamata olives, pitted and chopped
- 4 anchovy fillets, chopped
- 3 birds eye chillies, finely sliced
- good-quality olive oil
- 2 x 400g tins of italian tomatoes
- 1 cup rosa tomatoes
- ¼ cup cashew nuts, roasted
- handful fresh oregano, leaves picked and chopped
- salt and pepper
- ¼ cup cream
- 500g store-bought gnocchi
- knob of unsalted butter
- 1 cup ricotta cheese
- handful fresh basil, chopped, for garnishing

In a heavy-based saucepan, fry the garlic, capers, olives, anchovies and chilli in olive oil until the garlic is golden. Add the tomatoes, nuts and oregano, and bring to boil. Turn down the heat, season lightly and allow to simmer for 10 minutes. Stir in the cream and simmer for an additional 2 minutes.

In the meantime, cook the gnocchi in a pot of salted water. When the gnocchi rises to the surface, remove with a slotted spoon and toss with butter.

Crumble the ricotta into the sauce and stir to mix well. Serve the gnocchi in a bowl with a generous helping of sauce. Garnish with basil.

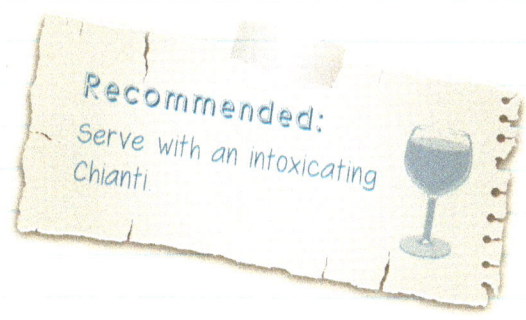

Recommended: Serve with an intoxicating Chianti.

The Back Flip

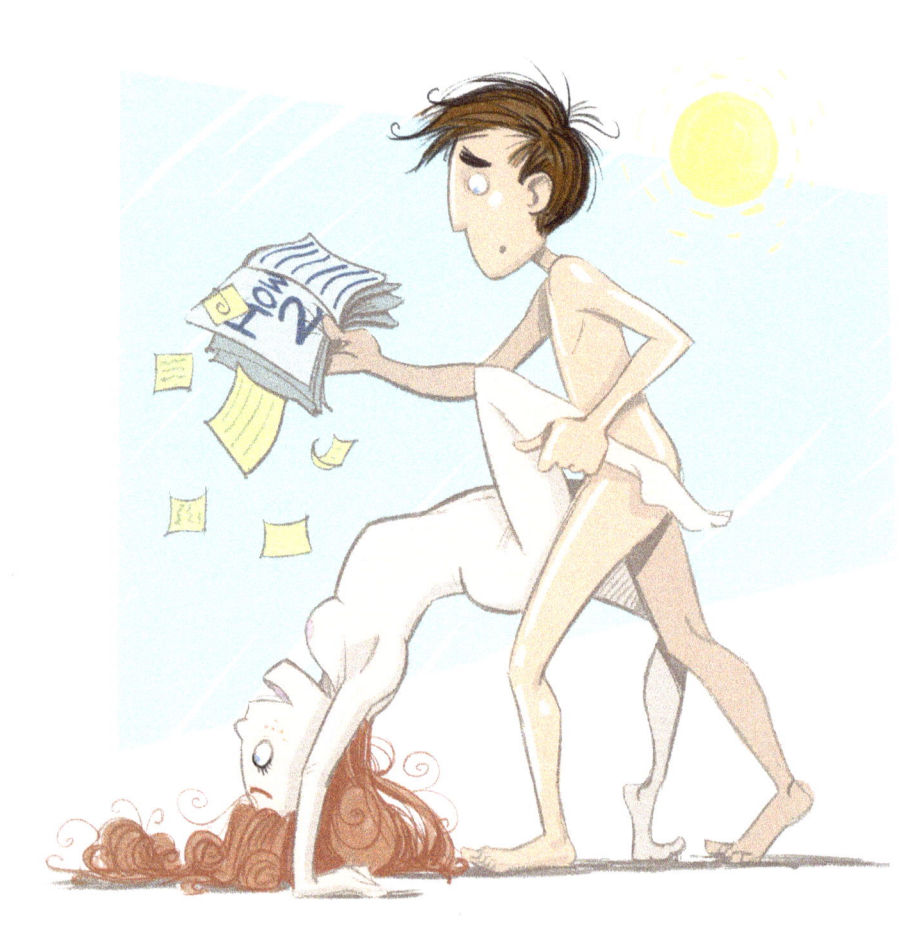

74

sweet and supple chick

easy

20 min

- 4 tbsp wholegrain mustard
- 2 tbsp honey
- 400g chicken thighs, skinless and deboned
- salt and pepper
- olive oil

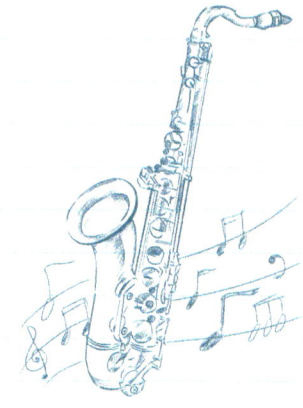

Put on some soothing jazz tunes to ease you into the mood.

Combine the mustard and honey in a shallow bowl. Take each thigh and roll it through the mustard mixture, generously coating each thigh. Season to taste. Bring a heavy-based pan to a medium heat and heat the olive oil. Fry each thigh until it is cooked through and opaque. Serve with mashed potato and your favourite vegetables.

Recommended:
Indulge in a wooded Chardonnay tasting of caramelised lemons... before you try the back flip.

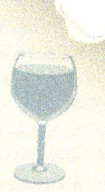

The Crack Filler

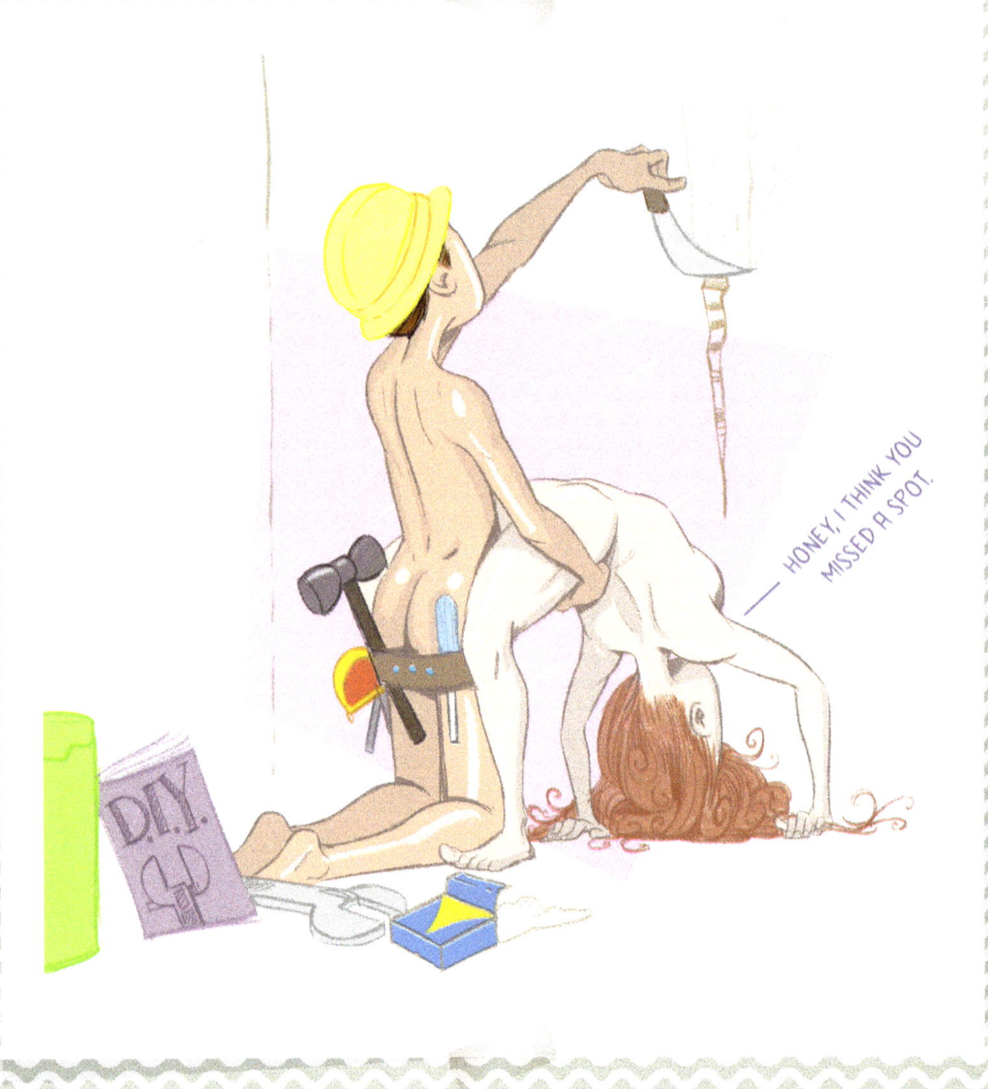

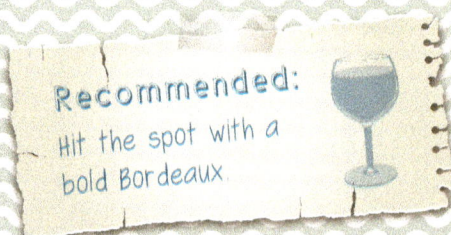

Recommended: Hit the spot with a bold Bordeaux.

beef shank bone

a lot of effort

> 60 min

CASSEROLE
- 2kg beef shank, on the bone
- olive oil
- 2 onions, peeled and chopped
- 2 fennel stems, chopped
- 2 parsnips, peeled and coarsely chopped
- 3 bay leaves
- 2 cups beef stock
- 400g tin crushed tomatoes
- 2½ cups dry red wine
- 8 sprigs thyme
- 4 sprigs rosemary
- 1 tbsp mustard powder

BASIL MASH
- 8 potatoes, peeled and halved
- ¼ cup milk
- knob of butter
- ¼ cup crème fraîche
- salt and pepper
- 4 sprigs basil, leaves picked

SIDE OF VEGETABLES
- 4 leeks
- 1 fennel bulb, sliced
- knob of butter
- salt and pepper

Coat the meat in olive oil and seal on a high heat in a large, cast-iron casserole. Take the casserole off the heat, remove the meat and place it on a wooden board to stand. Bring the casserole back to a medium heat, add a dash of olive oil, the vegetables and bay leaves. Cook the vegetables for 10 minutes or until slightly caramelised. Add the stock, tomatoes, wine and herbs, and bring the mixture to the boil. Rub the meat with mustard powder and then return it to the casserole. Cover and simmer for 6 hours, basting the meat twice. Before serving, remove the meat from the casserole and allow to stand for a few minutes.

To make the basil mash, boil the potatoes in salted water until soft and then drain. Put the potatoes back into the saucepan and add the milk, butter and crème fraîche. Mash to desired consistency. Season and stir in the basil.

To make the vegetables, gently sauté the leeks and fennel in butter until golden. Lightly season.

Serve the sumptuous meat on a bed of mash with the sautéed vegetables on the side. Pour the gravy and vegetables from the pot over the meat. This meal will keep you going for a few days!

The Side Saddle

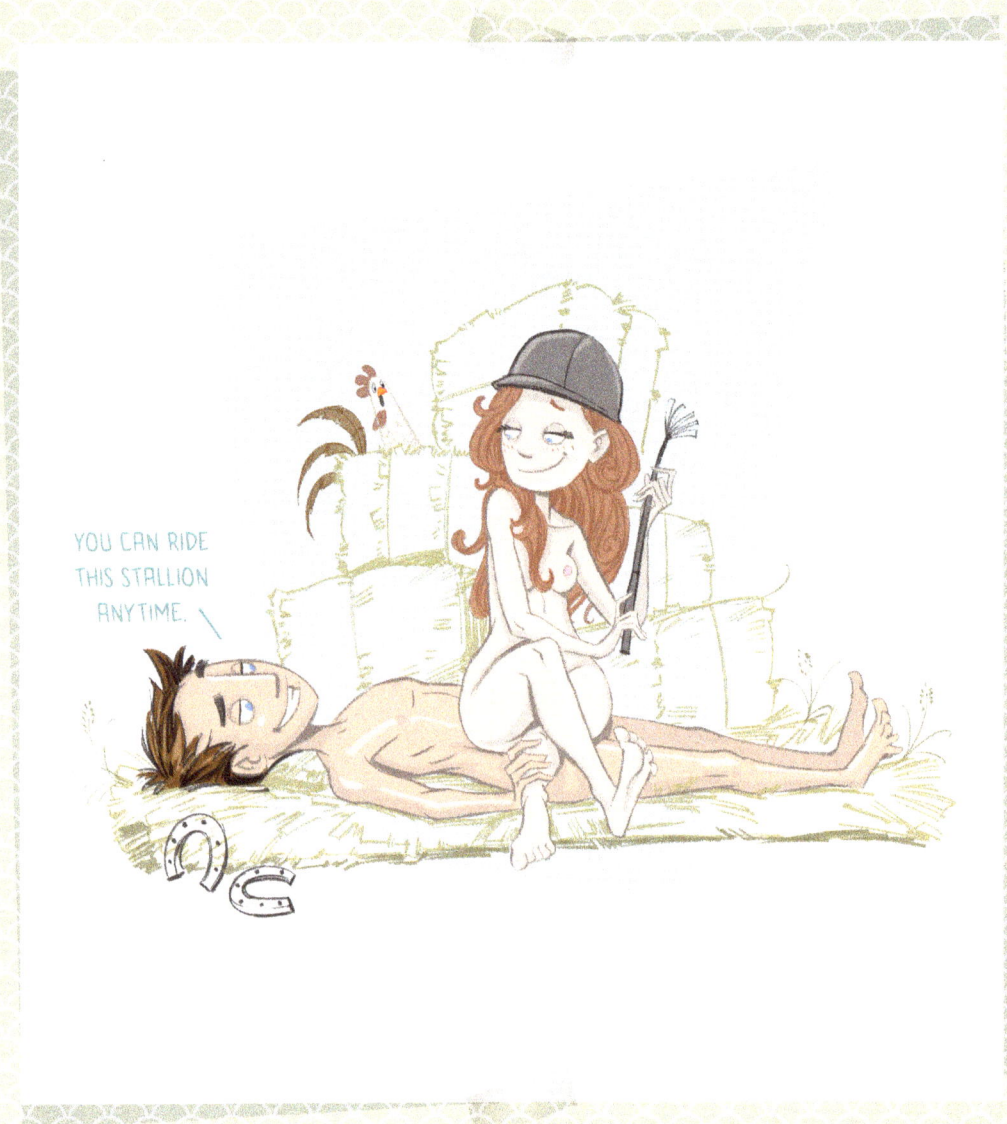

lusty langoustines

a little effort
>60 min

POTATO DISH

- juice and zest of 2 lemons
- sprig fresh thyme, chopped
- 1 cup vegetable stock
- 3 large potatoes, peeled and halved
- salt and pepper

SHELLFISH

- ¼ cup unsalted butter
- sprig fresh coriander, chopped
- 1 garlic clove, crushed
- 6 large langoustines, cleaned

Combine half the lemon zest and juice with the herbs and stock. Place the potatoes in an ovenproof dish and pour the lemon mixture over them. Season to taste. Pop into the oven and bake for 60 minutes at 190°C until the potatoes are soft, tossing from time-to-time.

Melt the butter in a microwave oven and add the remaining lemon juice and zest, coriander and garlic. Butterfly the langoustines and baste the flesh with the mixture. Put the langoustines over hot coals for about 8 minutes or until the colour has paled. The meat should peel easily from the shells. Serve the shellfish on a platter together with the fragrant potatoes.

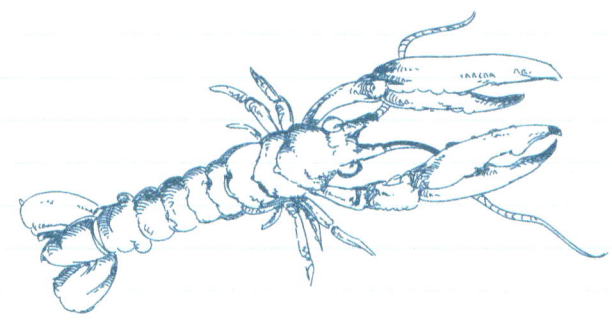

Recommended:
Such soft flesh balances well with a crisp and young Chenin Blanc.

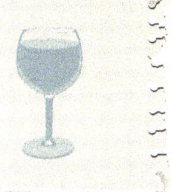

The Star Gazer

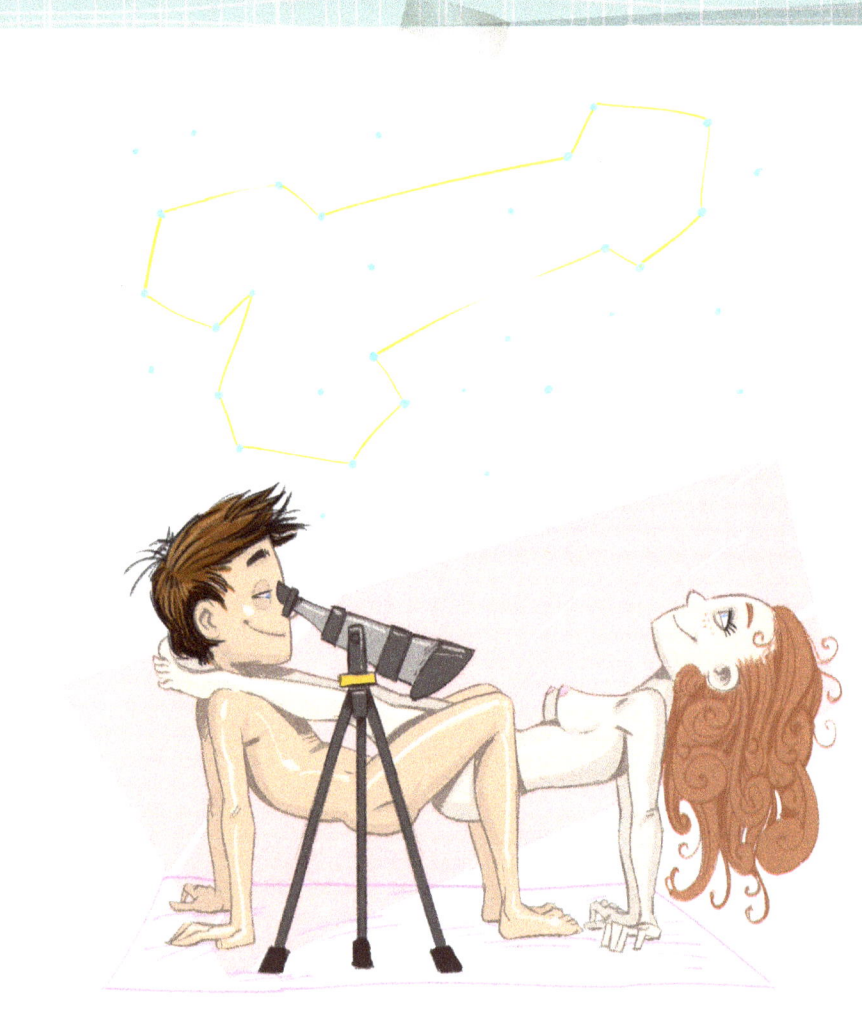

heavenly thighs

a little effort

\> 60 min

CRUMBED CHICKEN
- 400g chicken thighs, skinned and deboned
- sprig fresh thyme, leaves picked
- ½ cup breadcrumbs
- ¼ cup flour
- ¼ cup parmesan, grated
- salt and pepper
- ¼ cup olive oil
- ¼ lemon

POTATO SALAD
- ¼ cup edamame beans
- 6 baby potatoes, boiled and quartered
- sprig fresh parsley, chopped
- ¼ cup mayonnaise
- 2 tsp lemon juice
- salt and pepper to taste
- handful fresh coriander leaves

Boil the thighs in salted water for 5 minutes, drain and allow to cool slightly. In a bowl, mix together the thyme, breadcrumbs, flour, parmesan and seasoning. Dip each thigh into the olive oil and then into the breadcrumb mixture to coat. Place the thighs on a greased baking tray and put into the fridge for 10 minutes.

Remove the chicken from the fridge and bake in the oven for 20 minutes at 180°C until golden brown. Squeeze lemon juice over the chicken while it is still hot and serve with a tangy potato salad.

To make the potato salad, steam the beans for 5 minutes and allow to cool. In a small bowl, add the cooled potatoes, parsley, mayonnaise and lemon juice and mix. Season, top with the beans and garnish with a little coriander.

> **Recommended:**
> Delight in a spectacular view whilst enjoying a Sauvignon Blanc with citrus, lemon and fig flavours.

The Peeping Tom

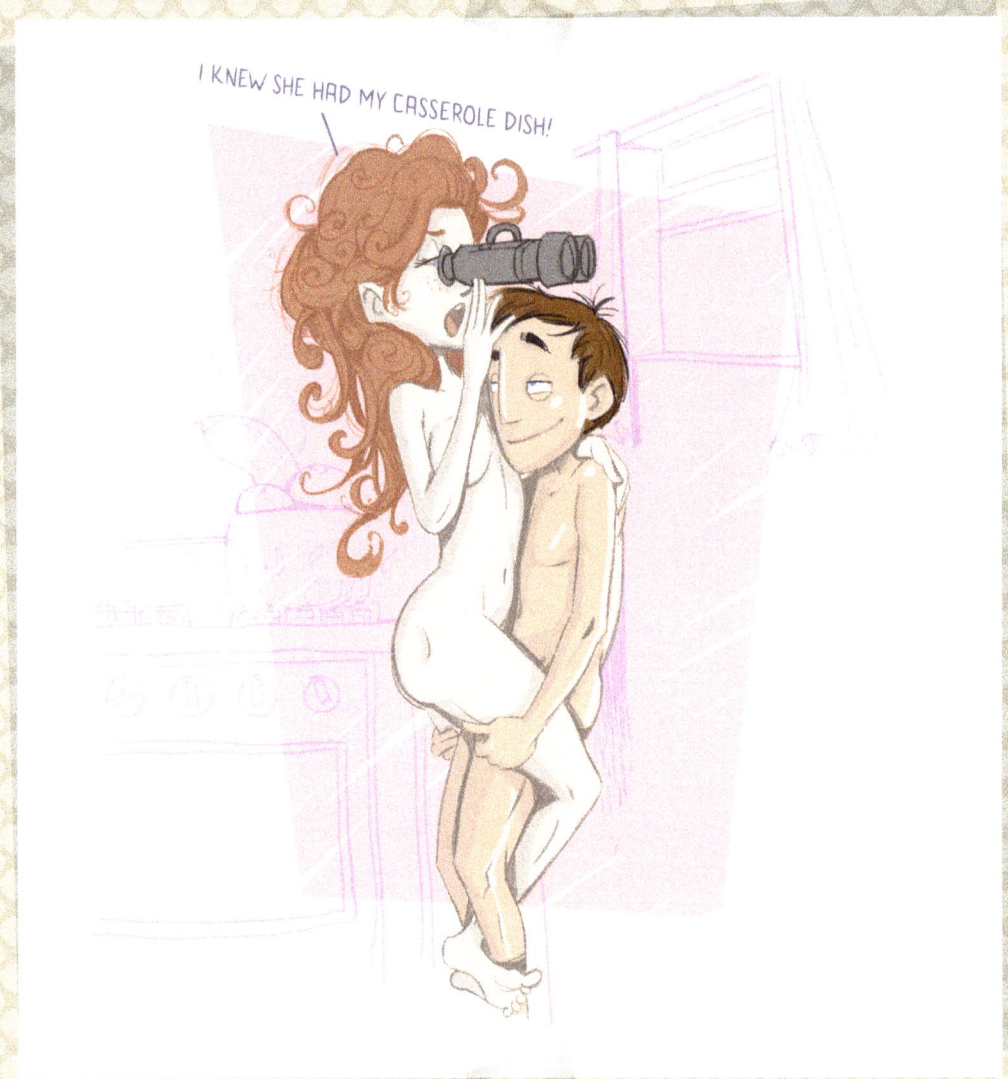

surreal casserole

easy
40 min

- 4 rashers streaky bacon
- 2 cups macaroni
- 2 cups ready-made béchamel sauce, heated
- 2 sprigs fresh parsley, chopped
- ¼ cup parmesan cheese, grated
- ground black pepper
- 2 sprigs fresh basil

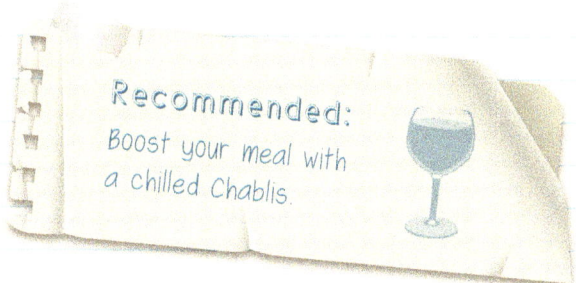

Recommended: Boost your meal with a chilled Chablis.

Grill the bacon until crispy and cut it into pieces. Cook the macaroni until al dente, drain and return it to the saucepan. Add the béchamel sauce, bacon and chopped parsley. Scoop the mixture into a casserole dish, sprinkle a layer of parmesan over the top and season to taste. Bake at 180°C for 20 minutes until deliciously crispy. Garnish with the basil leaves before serving.

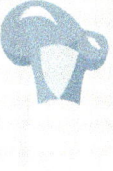

Tip: If you prefer to make your own béchamel sauce:
Dissolve 1 ½ tbsp of cornflour in ¼ cup cold milk. Pour the mixture into a saucepan and thicken over a medium heat, stirring constantly and gradually adding the remaining milk. Season with salt and pepper. Add the juice of ¼ lemon, a pinch of nutmeg and a pinch of ginger powder. Add 1 egg yolk and a tbsp of cream. Mix well and set aside.

THE OPERA

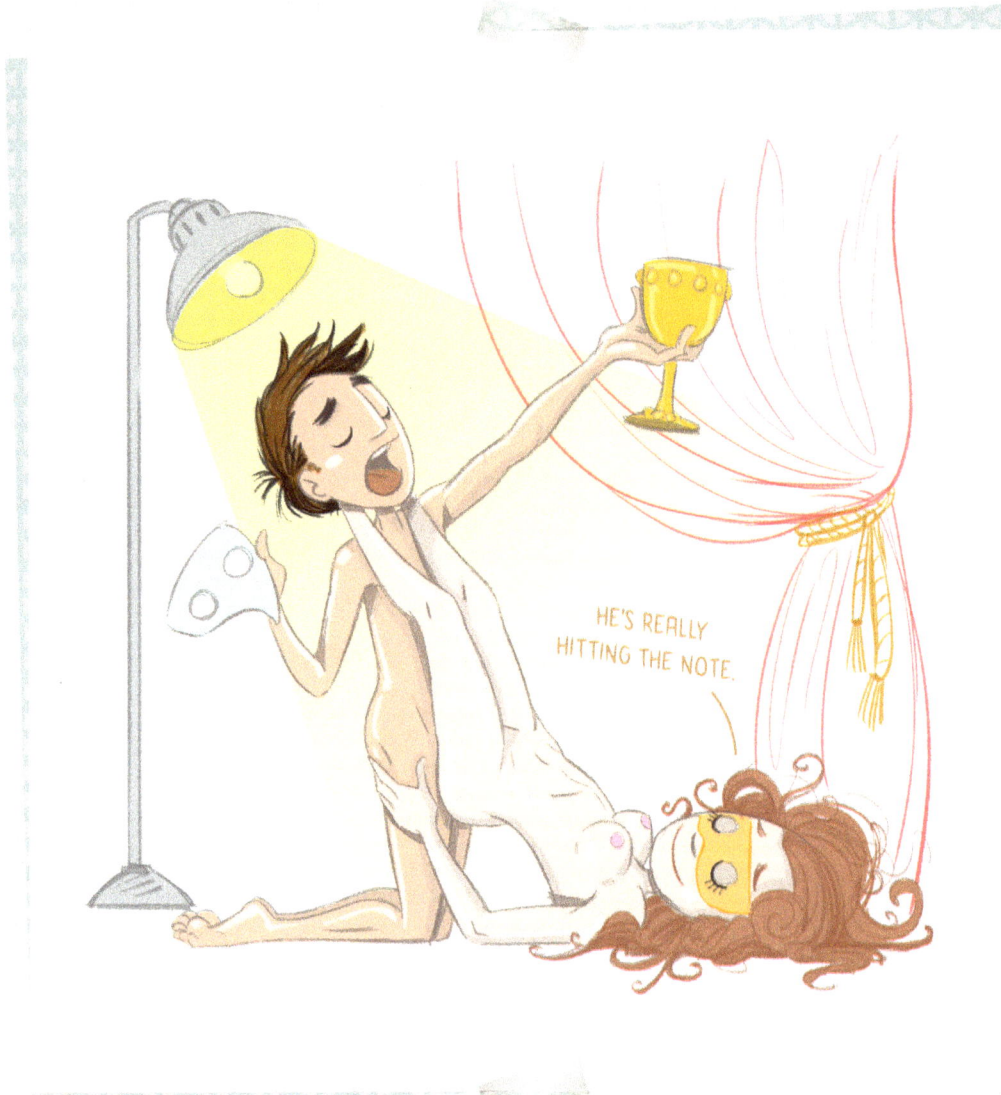

velvety tagliatelle

easy

25 min

- 2 cups cream
- ½ cup parmesan cheese, grated
- ¼ cup creamy gorgonzola cheese
- black pepper
- 2 handfuls broccoli florets
- 500g fresh tagliatelle
- 1 tbsp good-quality olive oil
- handful fresh chives, chopped, for garnishing

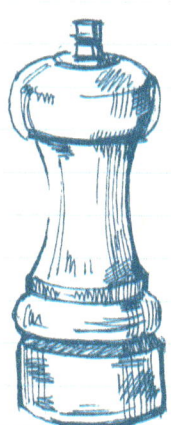

Place the cream in a large saucepan and bring to the boil. Lower the heat and simmer, reducing the cream to half. Add the cheese and season.

Bring a saucepan of salted water to the boil and blanch the broccoli until it is bright green. Remove from the heat, drain and rinse under cold water. Add the broccoli to the cheese mixture and stir gently to mix.

Bring a saucepan of salted water to the boil and cook the pasta to al dente. Remove from the heat, drain and put back into the saucepan. Toss the pasta with olive oil to prevent sticking. Add the cheese mixture, toss and serve garnished with the chives.

Recommended:
Impress her with your talent and a goblet of Viognier.

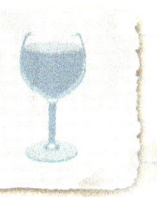

THE WINDY SHAFT

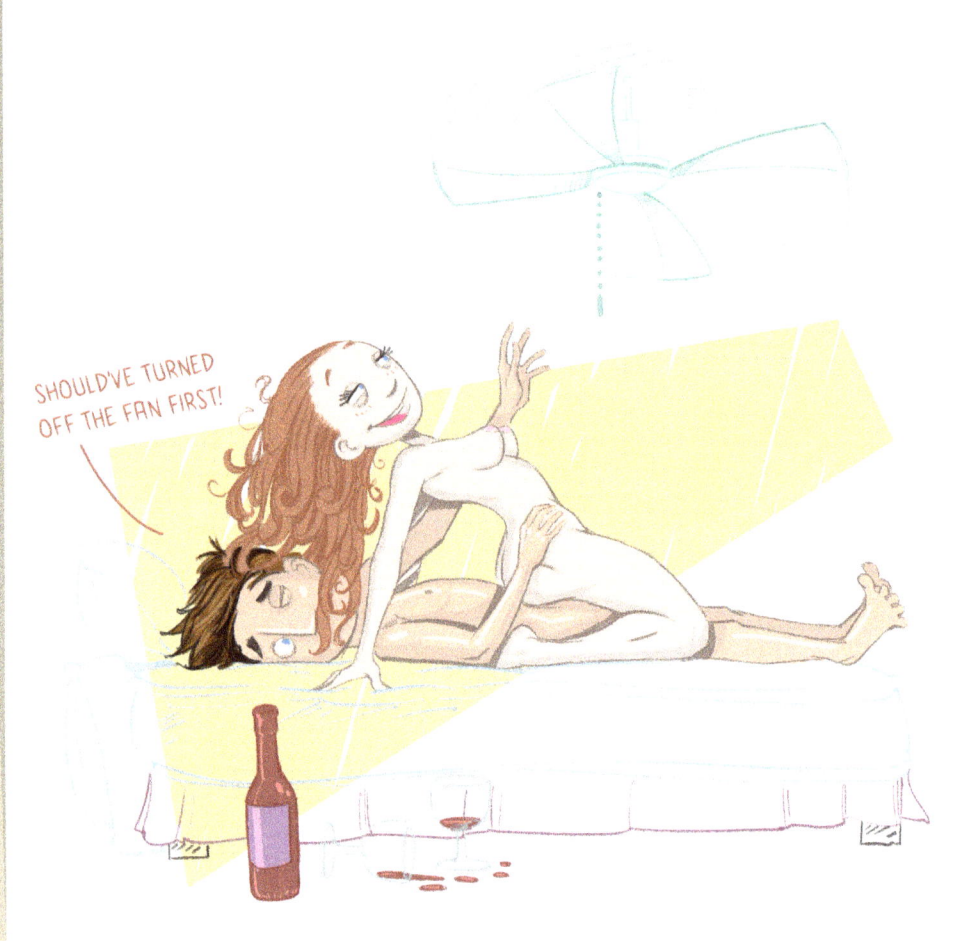

left-over wine

easy
> 60 min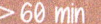

- ½ fillet of beef
- 2 cups red wine
- sprig fresh rosemary
- fresh green salad of mixed lettuce
- handful petit pois, steamed
- 2 carrots, sliced julienne
- sundried tomato reduction for drizzling
- sesame seeds, toasted
- 2 tsp tomato chilli jam
- ¼ cup emmenthal cheese, finely grated

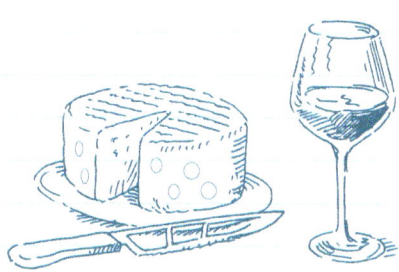
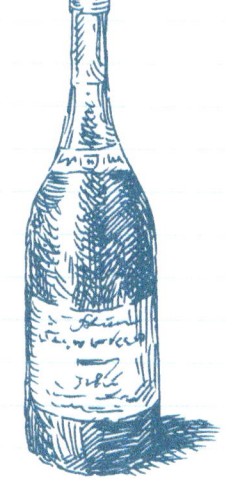

Marinate the meat in the wine and rosemary for 2 hours. Cook over hot coals to your preference, allow to cool and slice. On a serving platter, lay a bed of greens, petit pois and carrots. Add the sliced fillet and drizzle with the reduction. Sprinkle sesame seeds and top with tomato chilli jam. Finish off with a thin layer of grated cheese.

Recommended:
No harm in opening another bottle of wine! Try a red blend with a lingering, fruity aftertaste.

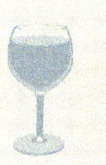

The Naughty Nurse

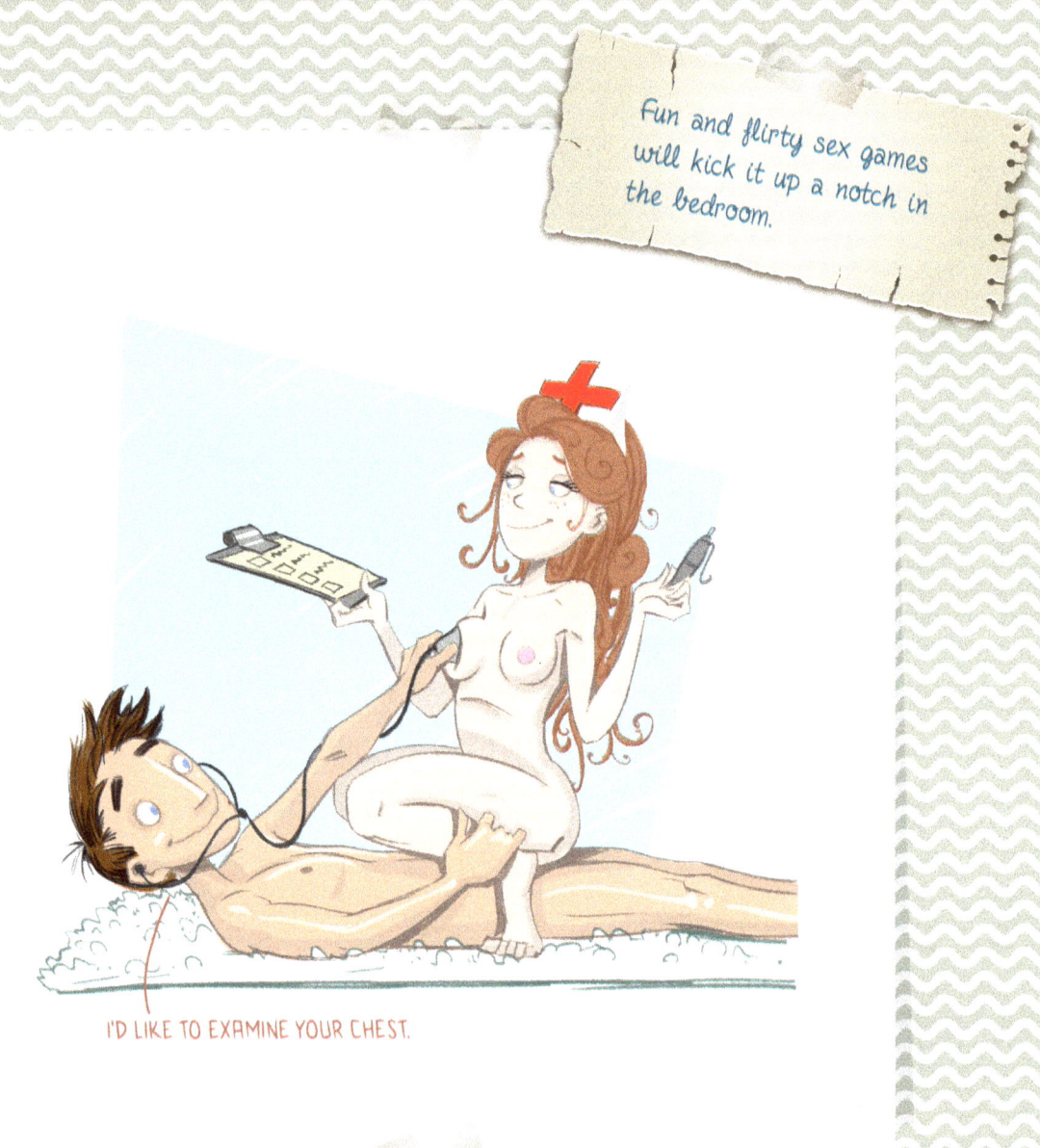

Fun and flirty sex games will kick it up a notch in the bedroom.

hot stuff lamb

easy
\> 60 min

- ½ leg of lamb, deboned and cubed
- 1 tbsp sunflower oil
- 1 tbsp red thai curry paste
- 400g tin coconut cream
- 3 curry leaves
- 1 tsp galangal
- 1 green chilli, coarsely chopped
- salt and pepper
- cornflour, if needed
- packet of pad thai noodles
- handful fresh coriander leaves, for garnishing

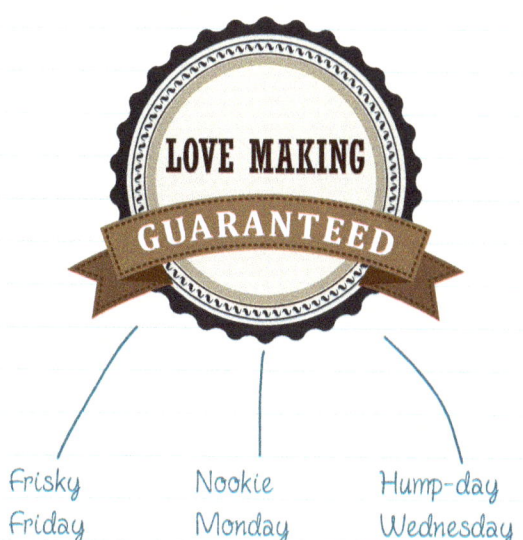

LOVE MAKING GUARANTEED

Frisky Friday   Nookie Monday   Hump-day Wednesday

Cook the lamb in oil on a medium heat to seal it. Add the curry paste and coat the lamb cubes. Add the coconut cream, curry leaves, spices and chilli. Bring the lamb to boil, and reduce to simmer for an hour. Season to taste and thicken the curry with cornflour if needed. Prepare the noodles as per instructions on the packet. Serve the noodles with a generous helping of lamb and garnish with coriander.

Recommended:
Tickle your senses with an intense and spicy Shiraz.

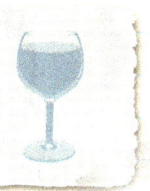

The Skipper

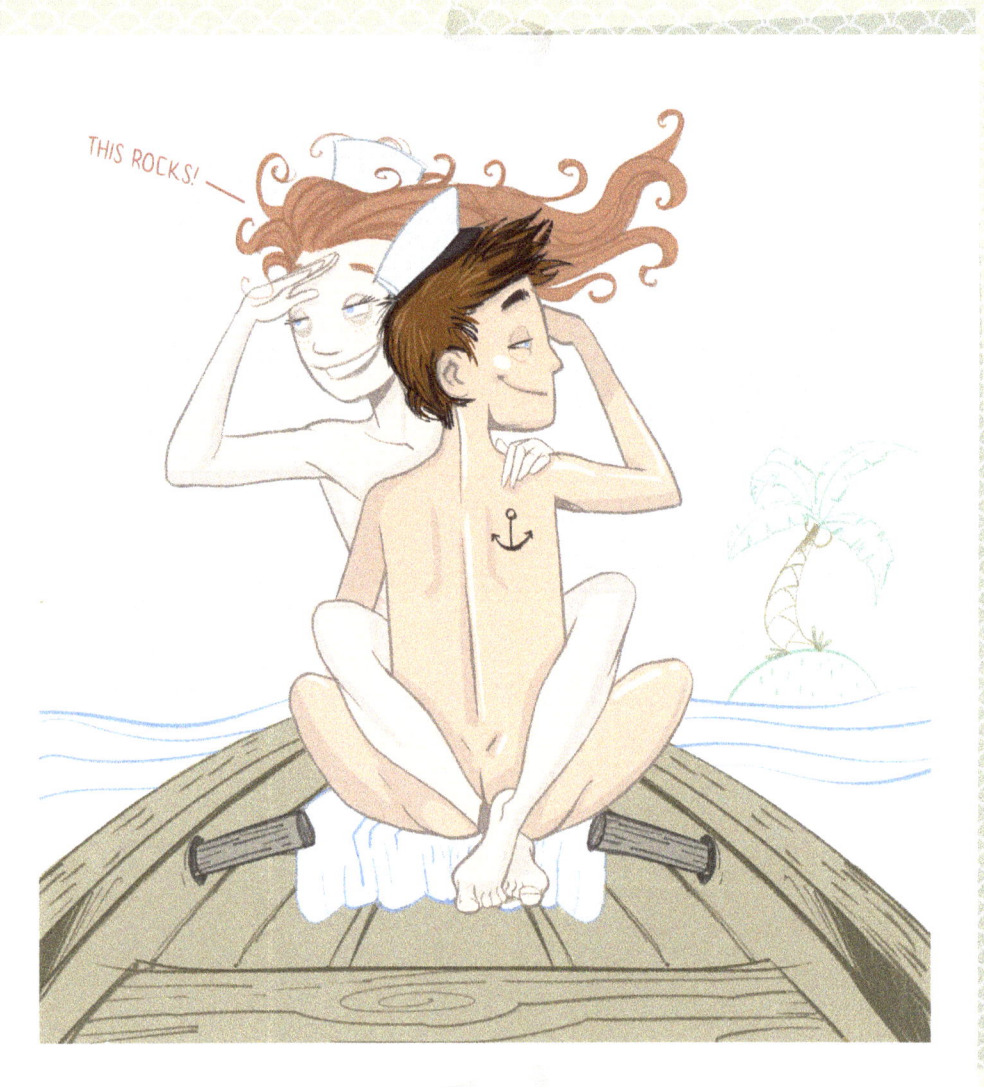

rocking kabeljou

a little effort

50 min

SALAD
- 1 cup wild brown rice
- 2 tbsp good-quality olive oil
- ½ cup dried cranberries
- ¼ cup pine nuts, toasted
- 1 salad onion, finely sliced
- sprig fresh mint, chopped
- ¼ cup lemon juice
- zest of ½ lemon
- 2 tsp dijon mustard
- sprig fresh basil, for garnishing

FISH PARCEL
- whole kabeljou, deboned and cleaned
- lemon butter, to rub
- sprig fresh fennel
- sprig fresh lemon thyme
- sprig fresh mint
- 1 lemon, sliced
- olive oil
- 1 lemon, quartered

To make the salad, cook the rice until tender, drain and rinse. Add the olive oil, cranberries, pine nuts, onion and mint, and toss well. To make a dressing, whisk the lemon juice, zest and mustard together and drizzle over the salad. Tear up the fresh basil to garnish.

Lay the fish out in some foil. Rub the lemon butter on the inside of the fish and stuff it with the fennel, thyme, mint and lemon slices. Brush the outside with olive oil. Wrap the foil around the fish to seal it well. Place your fish parcel over hot coals and allow the steam to cook it for about 20 minutes or until the fish is opaque. Serve with the salad and wedges of lemon.

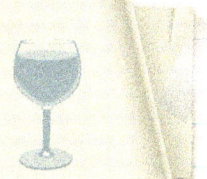

Recommended: Cook your fish out under the stars and select a racy Sauvignon Blanc to accompany it.

The Grower

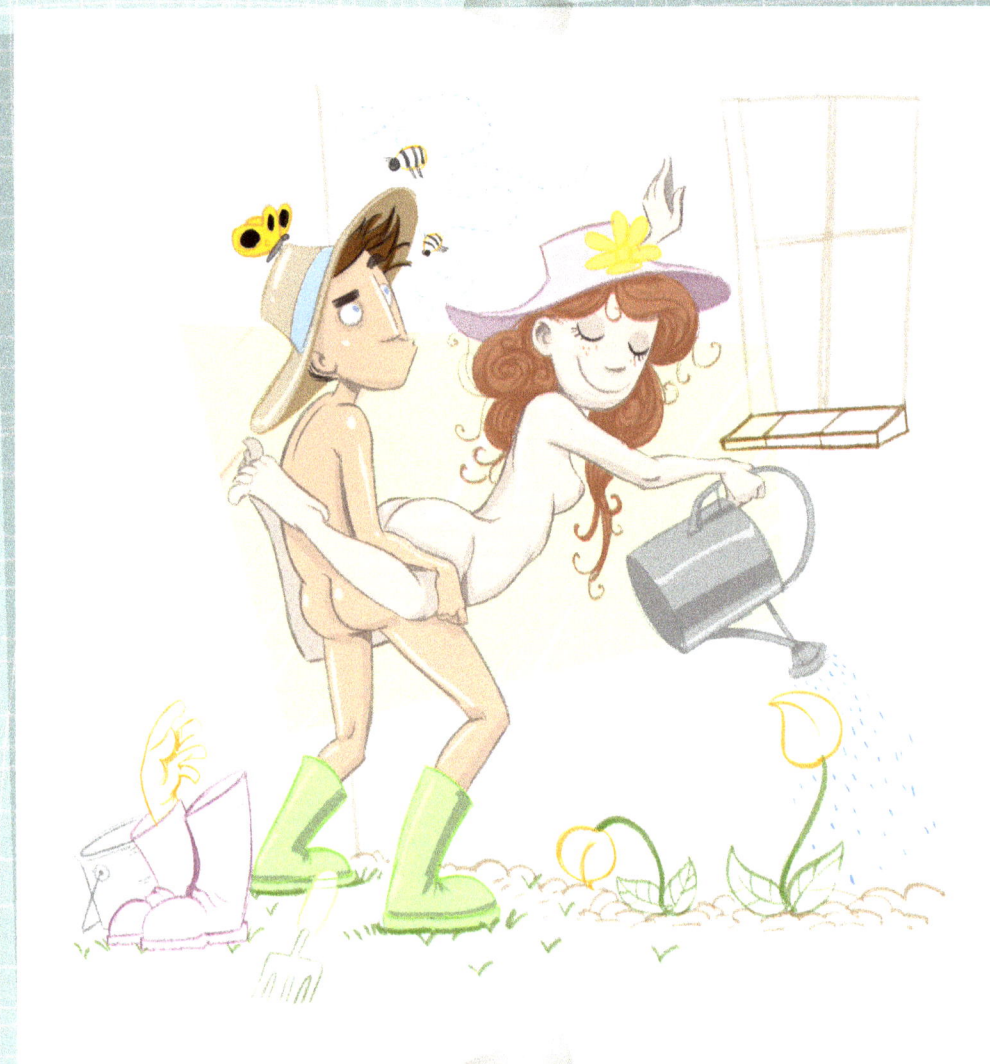

beefy wellies

a little effort

> 60 min

- 1 punnet portobello mushrooms, halved
- 1 clove garlic, crushed
- sprig fresh thyme, leaves picked
- 3 shallots, peeled and chopped
- olive oil
- fillet of beef
- salt and pepper
- 1 tbsp dijon mustard
- 6 slices prosciutto ham
- 1 packet ready-made puff pastry, defrosted
- 1 egg yolk, beaten
- 1 tsp coarse salt
- 2 sprigs thyme, for garnishing

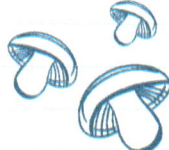

Blitz the mushrooms, garlic and thyme in a food processor. Fry the mushrooms dry until most of the moisture has been removed. Fry the shallots in a little oil until soft and set aside. Brush the fillet with olive oil, season and sear it to seal. Coat the fillet in a thin layer of mustard. Lay down the ham on a sheet of cling film, layer with the mushroom paste and place the fillet on top. Roll it tightly in the cling film and put in the fridge for 30 minutes. Remove the cling film and place the fillet on top of the pastry. Spoon the onion on top of the fillet, spreading it out. Wrap the fillet in the pastry and pinch the seams closed. Brush the pastry with egg, make criss-cross cuts on top, dust with salt crystals and pop in the oven at 200°C for 20 minutes or until golden brown. Allow to rest before serving. Garnish with thyme.

Recommended:
You can't beat a beef wellie served with an intense and fruity Cabernet Sauvignon.

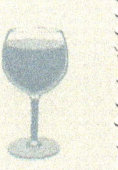

The Greek Dip

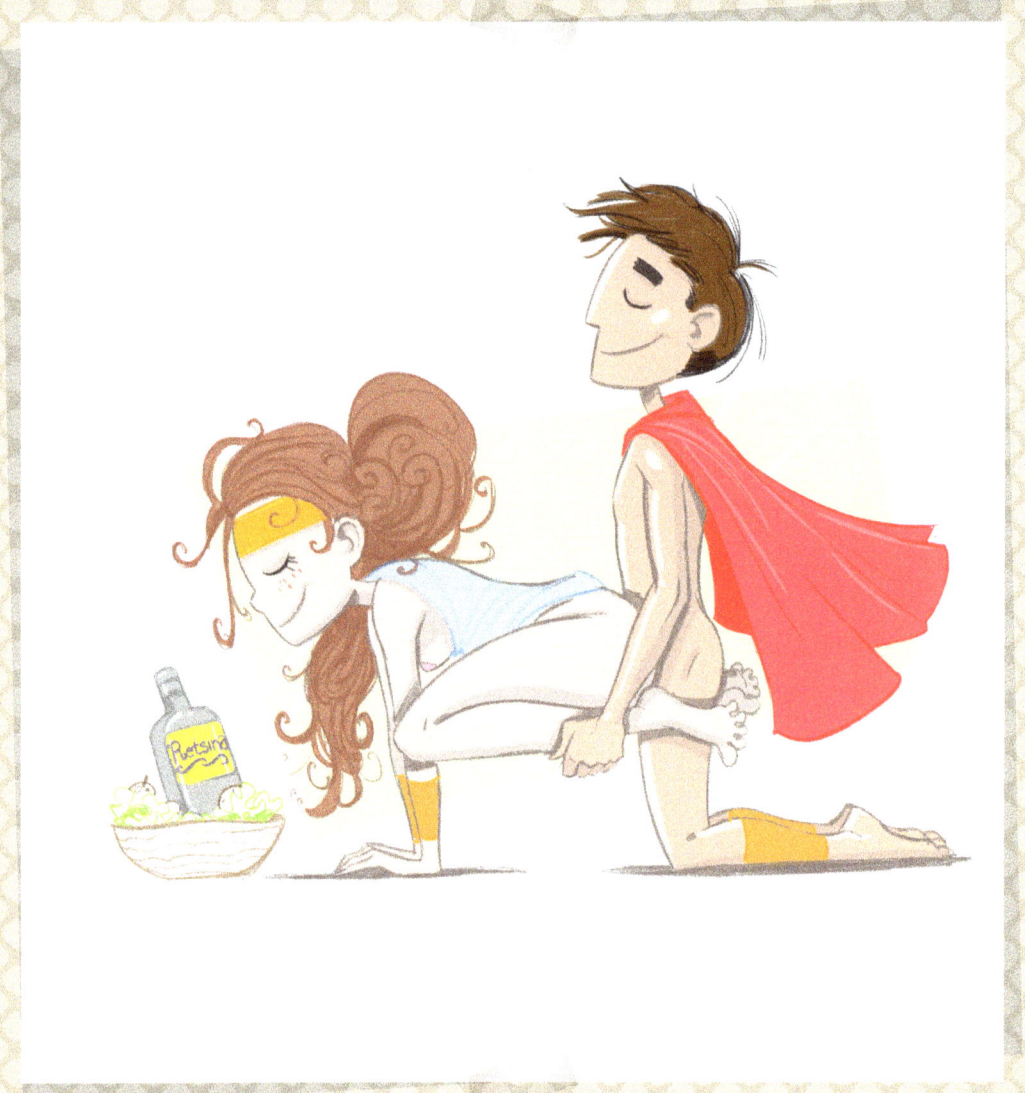

greek-style kebabs

a little effort

> 60 min

- 1 cup greek yogurt
- 1 tsp crushed garlic
- juice of 1 small lemon
- zest of ½ lemon
- handful fresh oregano, chopped
- handful fresh parsley, chopped
- salt and pepper
- 300g chicken breasts, cut into large chunks
- 6 bay leaf stems
- 1 head of cos lettuce, shredded
- 2 lemon wedges, for serving

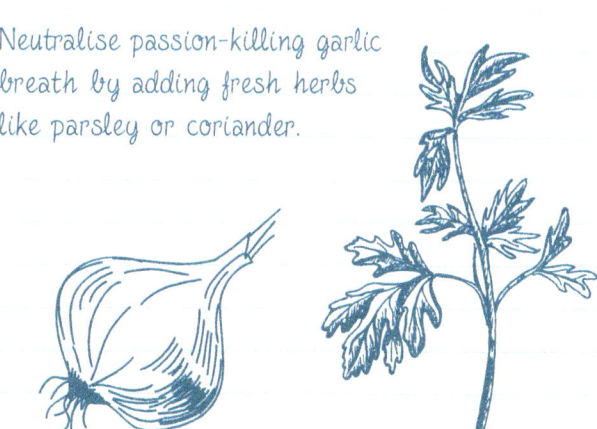

Neutralise passion-killing garlic breath by adding fresh herbs like parsley or coriander.

Mix the yogurt, garlic, lemon juice, zest and herbs together. Season to taste. Toss the chicken chunks in the mixture to coat each piece well. Cover and put in the fridge to marinate for 2 hours. Thread the chicken chunks onto the stems. Cook over hot coals until brown and cooked through but still tender. Turn and baste regularly. Warm the remaining yogurt sauce in a small saucepan. Serve the kebabs on a bed of cos lettuce with the lemon wedges and yogurt sauce.

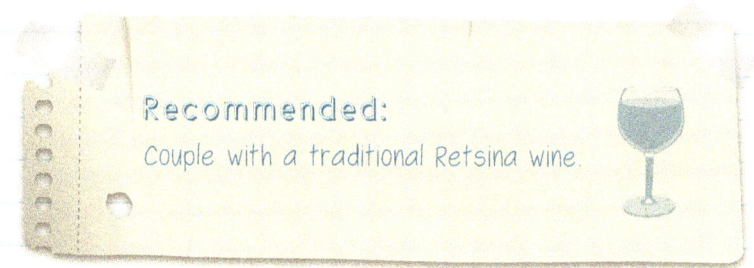

Recommended:
Couple with a traditional Retsina wine.

THE SWINGER

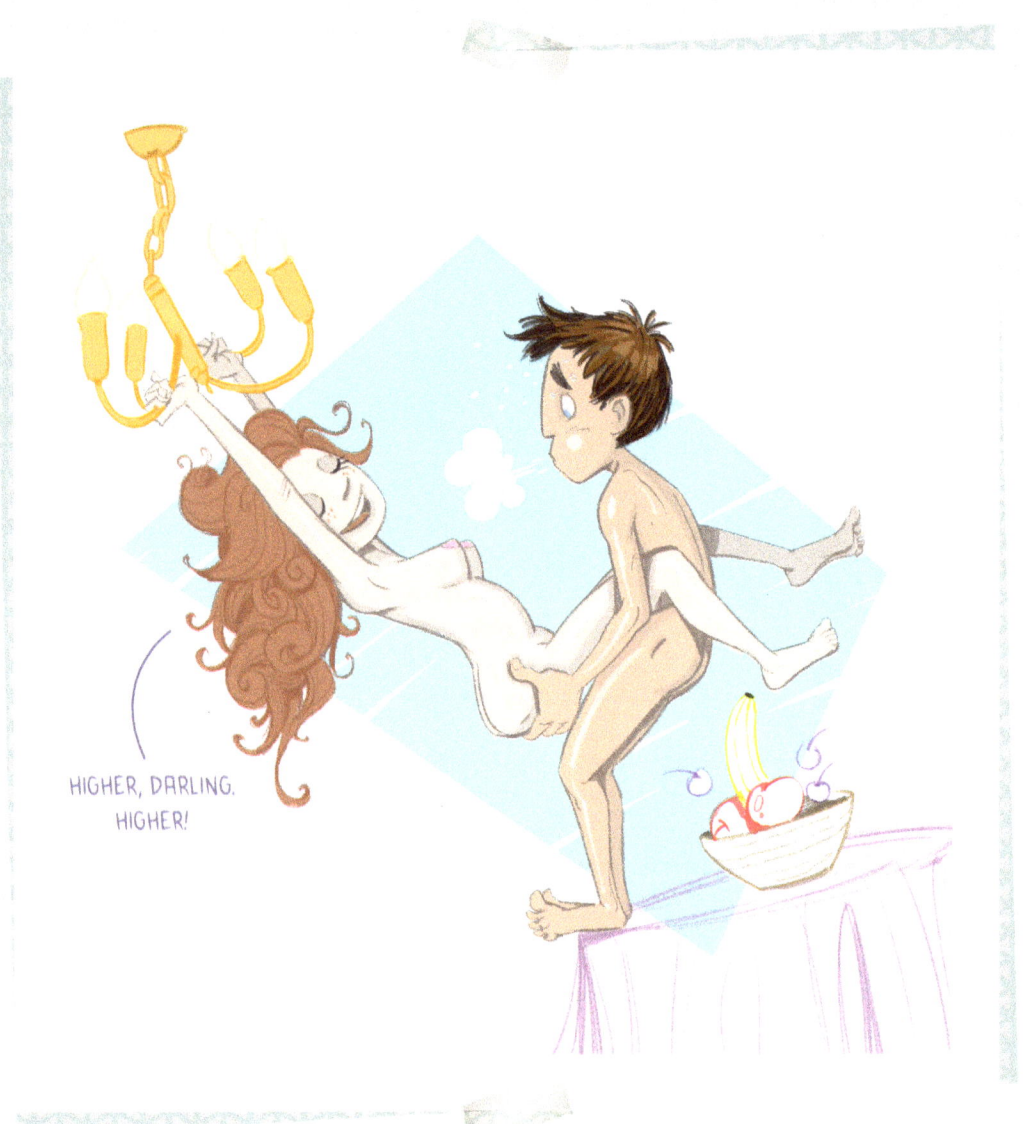

succulent plum fillet

a little effort

> 60 min

OSTRICH FILLETS
- 3 fresh plums, stones removed
- 2 tbsp sweet soy sauce
- 1 cup red wine
- 2 green chillies, chopped
- 4 cloves
- ostrich fillet, cut as medallions

SIDE OF VEGETABLES
- handful green beans
- 1 shallot, peeled and cut into thin slices
- 2 new potatoes, peeled and cubed
- 1 tbsp butter
- salt and pepper

Blitz the plums, soy sauce and red wine in a food processor. Put the mix, chillies and cloves in a bowl. Add the ostrich medallions to the mix and leave in the fridge to marinate for at least 3 hours. Grill the fillet on a high heat until cooked but slightly pink inside, basting regularly. Steam the vegetables and potatoes, melt in the butter and season to taste. Plate up the fillet and vegetables, and enjoy.

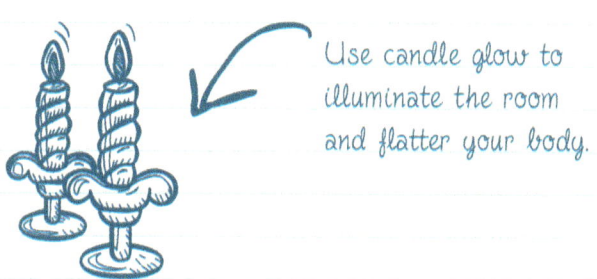

Use candle glow to illuminate the room and flatter your body.

Recommended:
Hold on tight and have a full-bodied Malbec ready on landing.

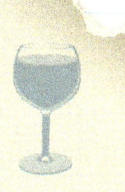

Notes

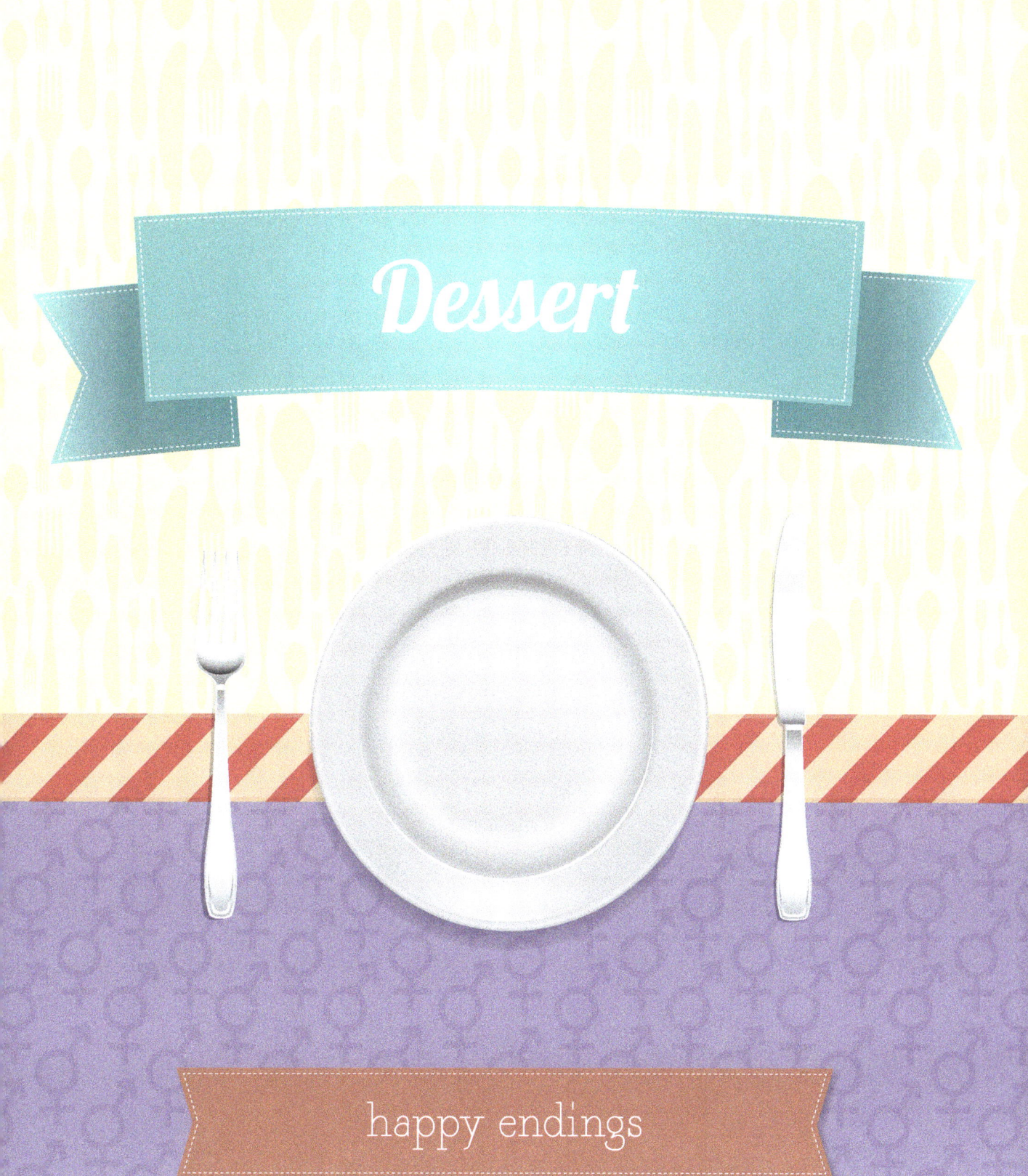

The Bungee Jumper

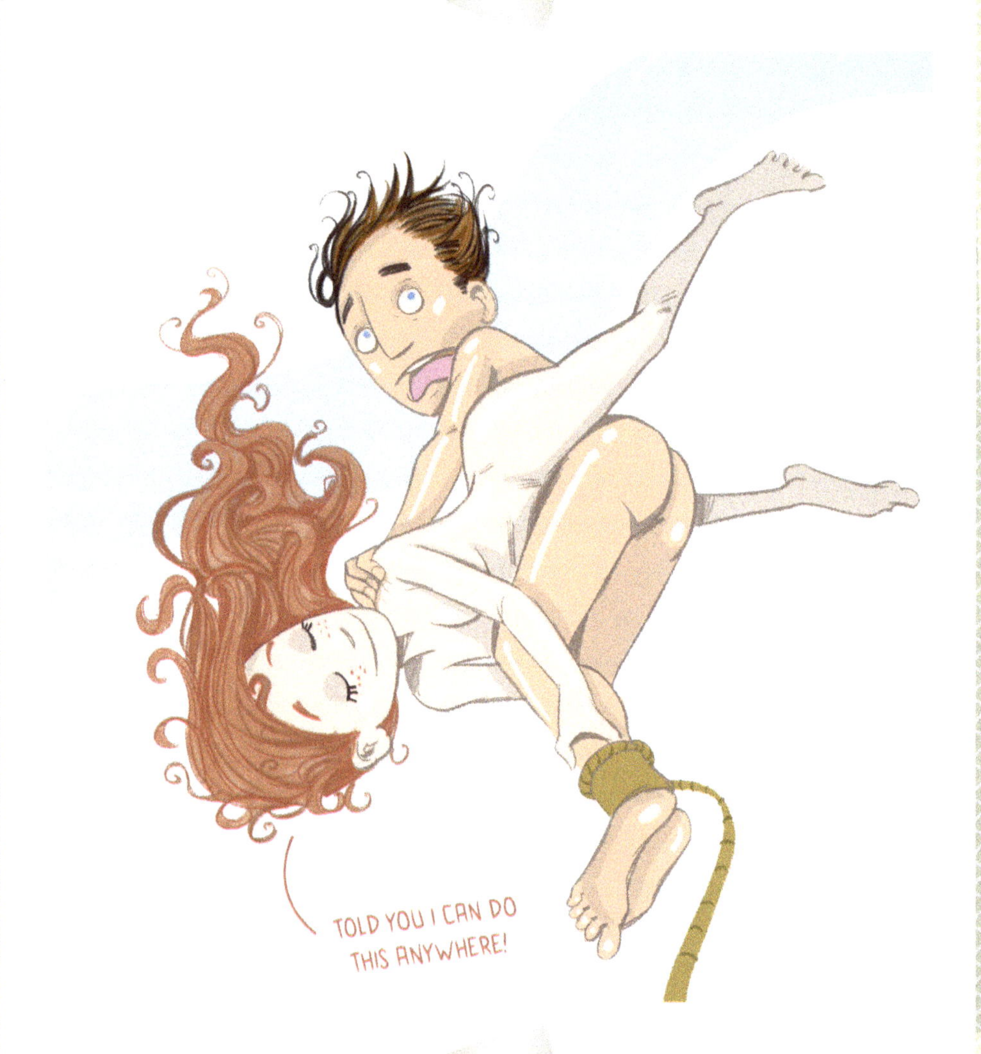

Told you I can do this anywhere!

A sugar rush will spark adventure and randiness anywhere...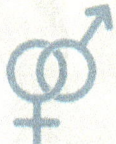

drunken pavlova

a little effort
> 60 min

- 2 cups raspberries
- 1 cup pale rum
- 6 egg whites, at room temperature
- 1 cup castor sugar
- 1 vanilla pod, seeds removed
- 1 tsp white wine vinegar
- 3 tbsp cocoa powder
- ¼ cup good-quality dark chocolate, chopped
- 2 cups whipping cream
- icing sugar, for dusting
- sprig fresh mint, leaves picked, for garnishing

Soak the raspberries in the rum overnight.

Beat the egg whites with an electric beater until you have firm and silky peaks. Turn the beater down to low and gradually add the sugar. Gently fold in the vanilla, vinegar, cocoa and chocolate bits. Line a large baking tray with wax paper and heap the meringue mixture onto the tray in a rough circle with a diameter of about 20cm. Smooth the sides and top with the back of a spoon. Bake at 160°C for an hour or until the outside shell is crisp but the centre is still soft to touch. Turn off the oven and allow the meringue to cool in the oven. Remove when cool.

Whip the cream to form soft peaks and spread crudely over the meringue. Drain the raspberries and scatter over the cream. Lightly dust with the icing sugar and garnish with a few mint leaves. Use the remaining raspberry sauce to drizzle around the plate when serving.

Recommended:
Take your dessert with a drunken Irish coffee.

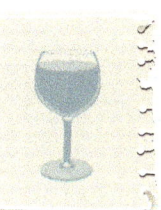

The Tattoo

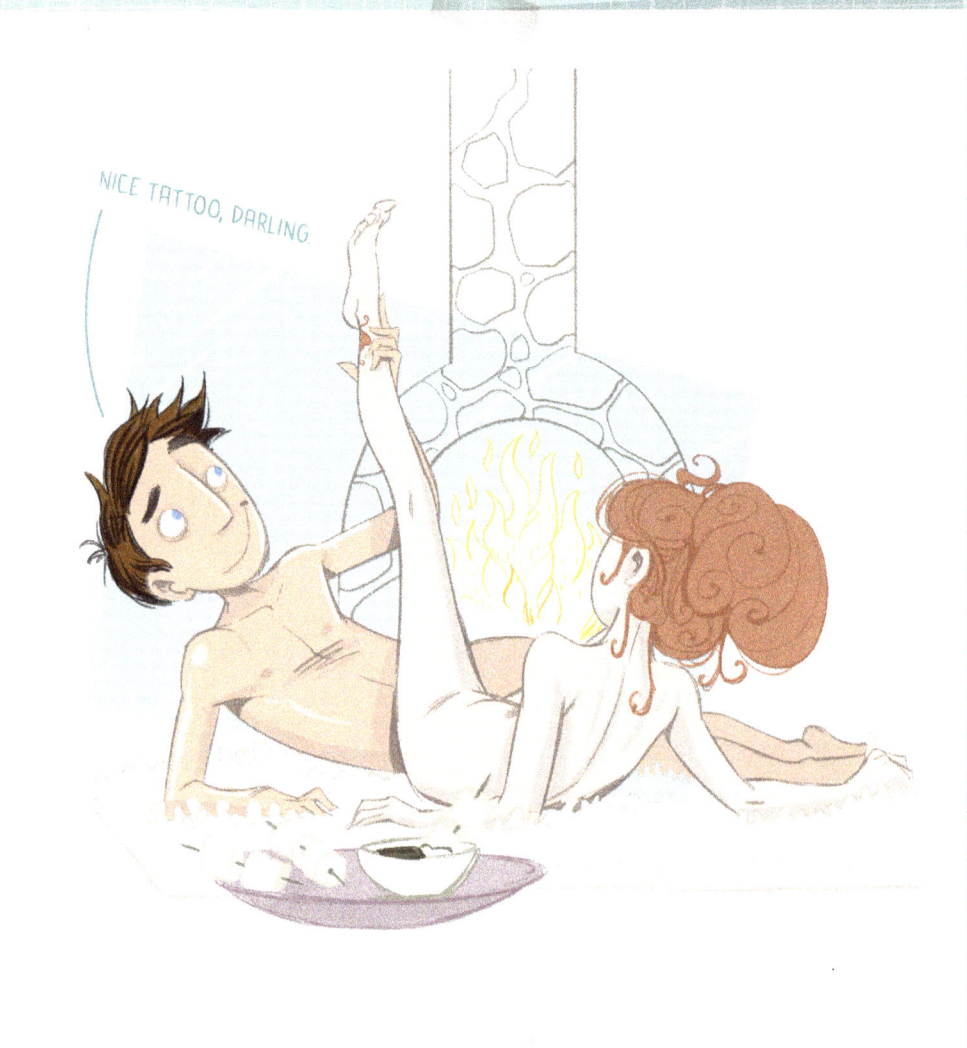

seductive marshmallows

easy
20 min

- 400g marshmallows
- 200g good-quality dark chocolate, chopped
- ½ cup full cream milk
- ¼ cup double thick cream
- 2 tbsp unsalted butter
- 1 tbsp grand marnier
- ½ cup toasted almonds, chopped

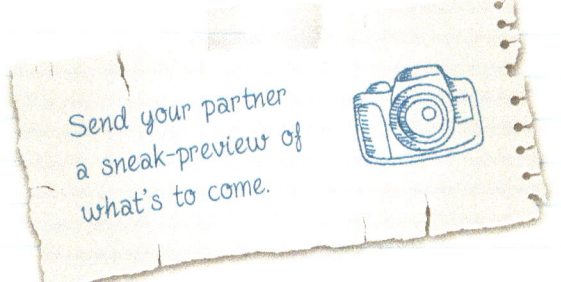

Send your partner a sneak-preview of what's to come.

Thread two marshmallows at a time onto a skewer and set aside on a platter.

Put the chocolate, milk, cream and butter into a saucepan and heat gently, stirring occasionally. When the butter has melted and the sauce is smooth, stir in the Grand Marnier. Serve the sauce in a dipping bowl and the almonds in a second bowl.

Toast the marshmallows on a fire and allow to cool slightly. Dip into the sauce followed by a roll in the almond flakes.

Recommended:
Enjoy alongside a toasty fire and with a tot of Muscadel.

The Ice Dancer

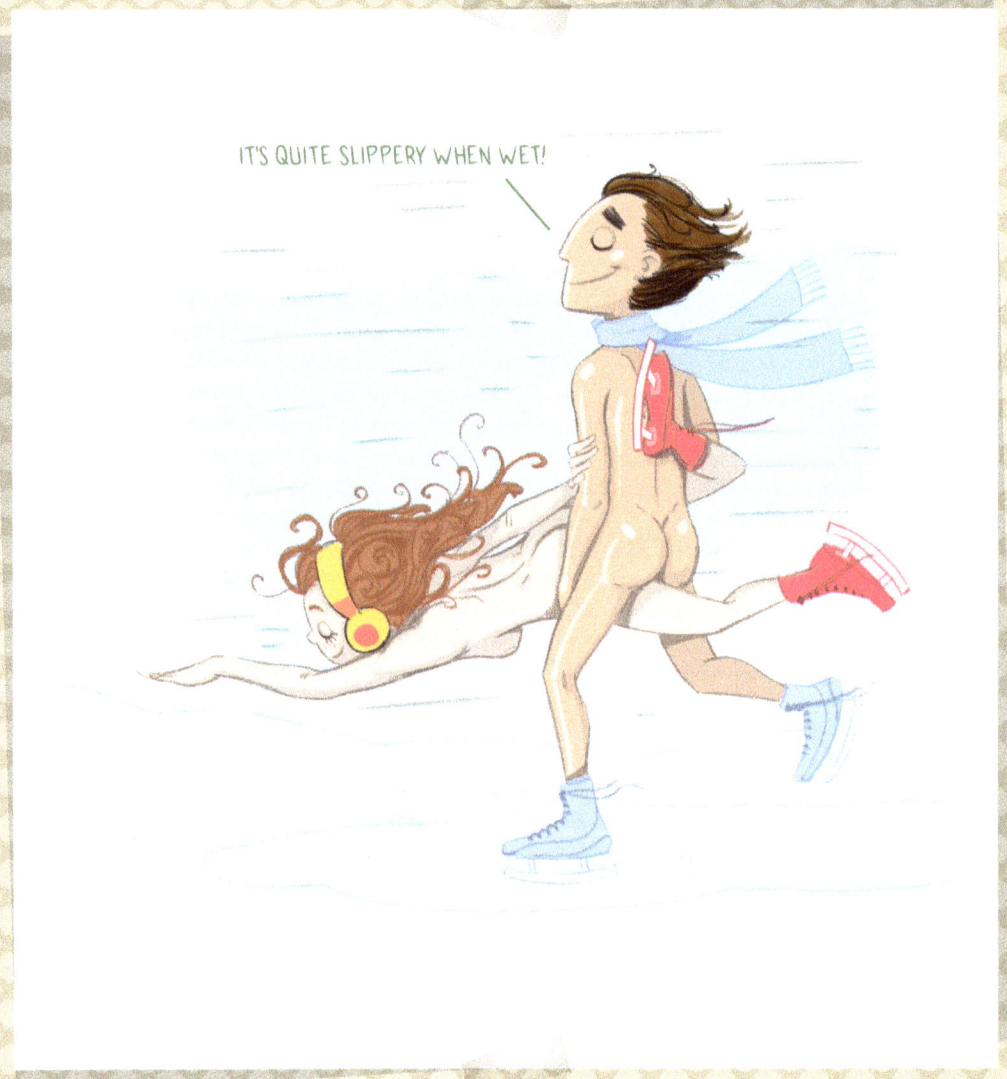

frozen kahlua cake

easy
> 60 min

- 2 litres good-quality coffee ice cream, softened
- ¼ cup kahlua coffee liqueur
- handful hazelnut wafers, broken into chips
- ½ cup maraschino cherries, drained and stalks removed
- 200g dark chocolate
- 1 tsp instant coffee
- ¼ cup roasted hazelnuts, finely chopped
- handful maraschino cherries for decorating

Line a loaf tin with cling wrap so that the plastic overlaps all sides. Empty the coffee ice cream into a mixing bowl and stir in the liqueur, wafer chips and cherries. Scrape the ice cream mixture into the tin, flattening into the mould with the back of a spoon. Freeze overnight.

In a double-boiler, melt the chocolate and coffee together. Remove the ice cream from the freezer and lift it from the tin using the cling wrap as handles. Turn it over onto a serving plate and discard the plastic. Slowly pour the melted chocolate over the ice cream cake, allowing it to drip down the sides. Sprinkle an even layer of the hazelnuts over the chocolate topping and return to the freezer for 10 minutes. Stand at room temperature for 5 minutes before serving, and decorate with the cherries.

Recommended:
Warm each other up and enjoy with a B52 cocktail.

The Learner Driver

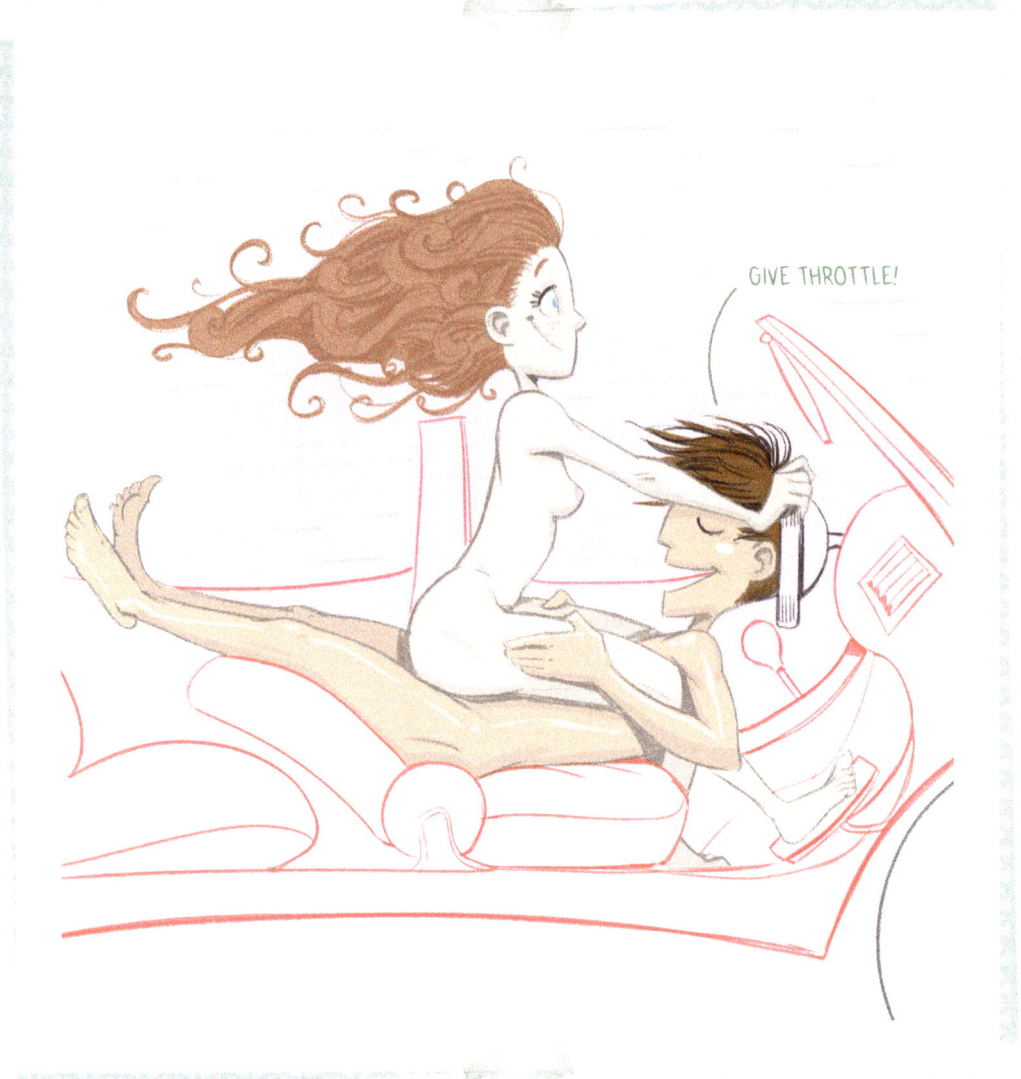

travelling chocolate pots

easy

15 min

- ½ cup brown sugar
- ½ tsp baking powder
- ½ cup cake flour
- 3 tbsp cocoa
- 2 eggs
- ⅓ cup milk
- ⅓ cup oil
- ¼ cup toasted macadamia nuts, chopped
- 6 large squares dark mint chocolate
- sprig fresh mint, for garnishing

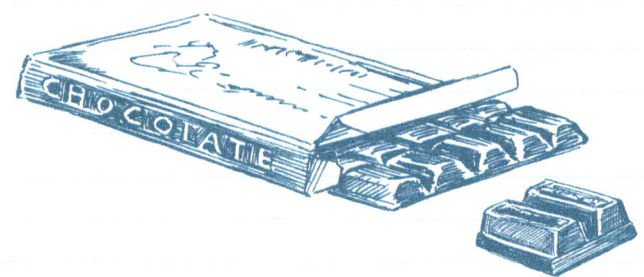

In a bowl combine the sugar, baking powder, flour and cocoa. Whisk in the eggs, milk and oil. Mix in the nuts ensuring all the ingredients are well combined. Divide the chocolate mixture into oven-proof espresso mugs. Slide one square of chocolate into the middle of each mug and pop into the microwave oven for about 2 minutes. Allow to cool and garnish with mint.

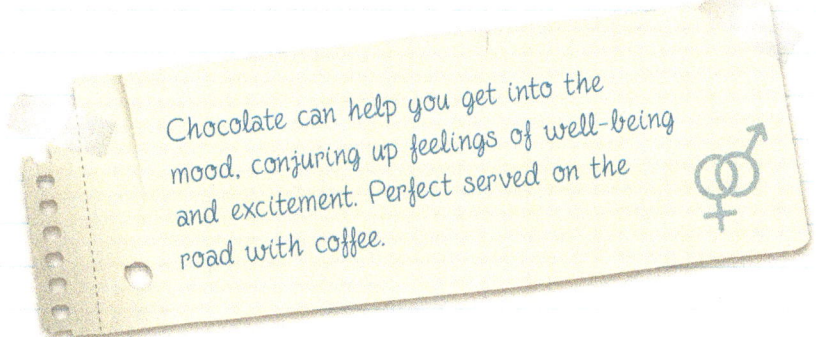

Chocolate can help you get into the mood, conjuring up feelings of well-being and excitement. Perfect served on the road with coffee.

The Babymaker

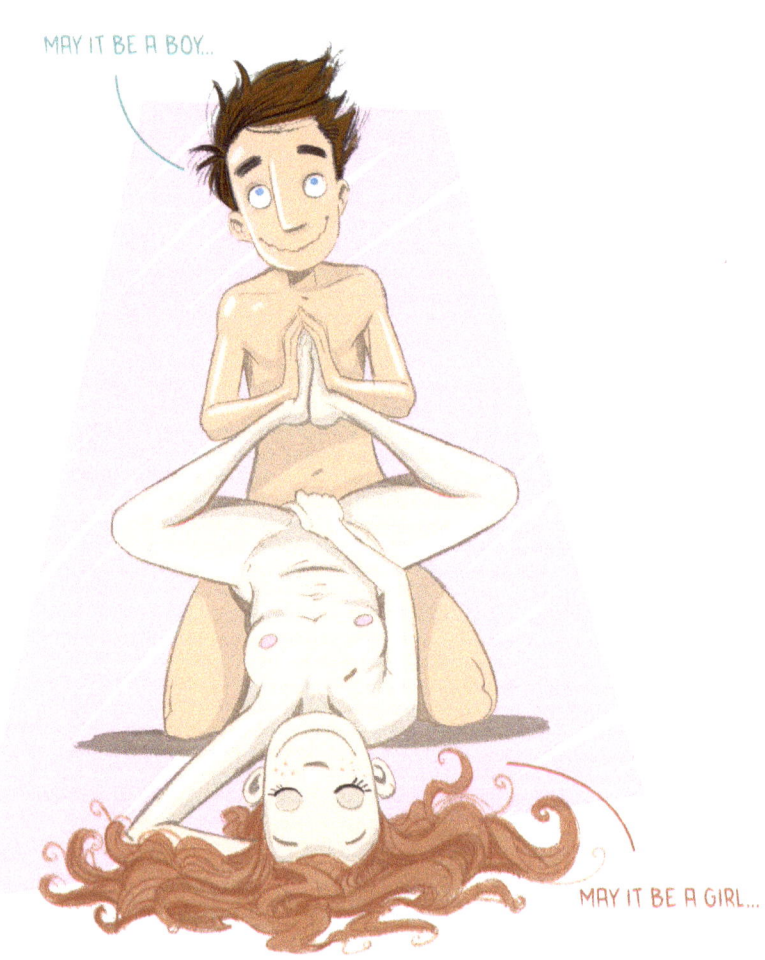

celebration jelly

easy
\> 60 min

- 1 cup strawberries, stalks removed and quartered
- 1 cup blueberries
- 750ml pink champagne
- ½ cup castor sugar
- 2 tbsp gelatine
- ¼ cup hot water
- sprig fresh mint, for garnishing

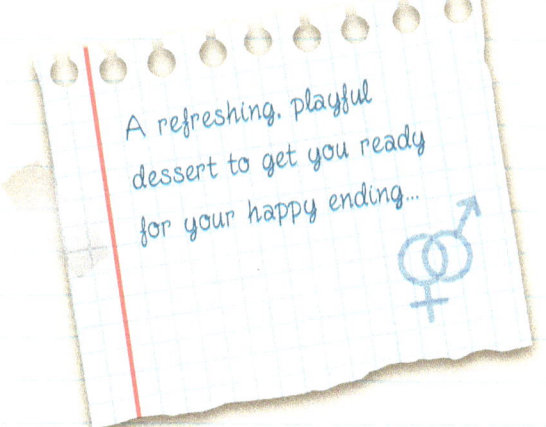

A refreshing, playful dessert to get you ready for your happy ending...

Prepare decorative, heat-proof glasses by arranging the berries on the base and up the sides of the glass. Combine the Champagne and sugar in a saucepan and slowly heat the mixture, stirring gently until the sugar dissolves. Remove from the heat. Sprinkle gelatine over the hot water and whisk briskly with a fork until it dissolves. Add the gelatine mixture to the Champagne mixture and stir to combine. Pour the Champagne mixture slowly into the glasses and allow to cool. Place in the fridge for a few hours or overnight to set. Garnish with mint when serving.

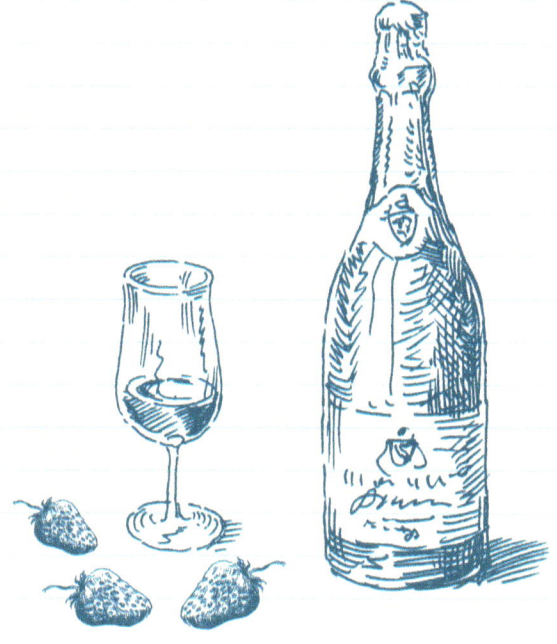

The Multi-Tasker

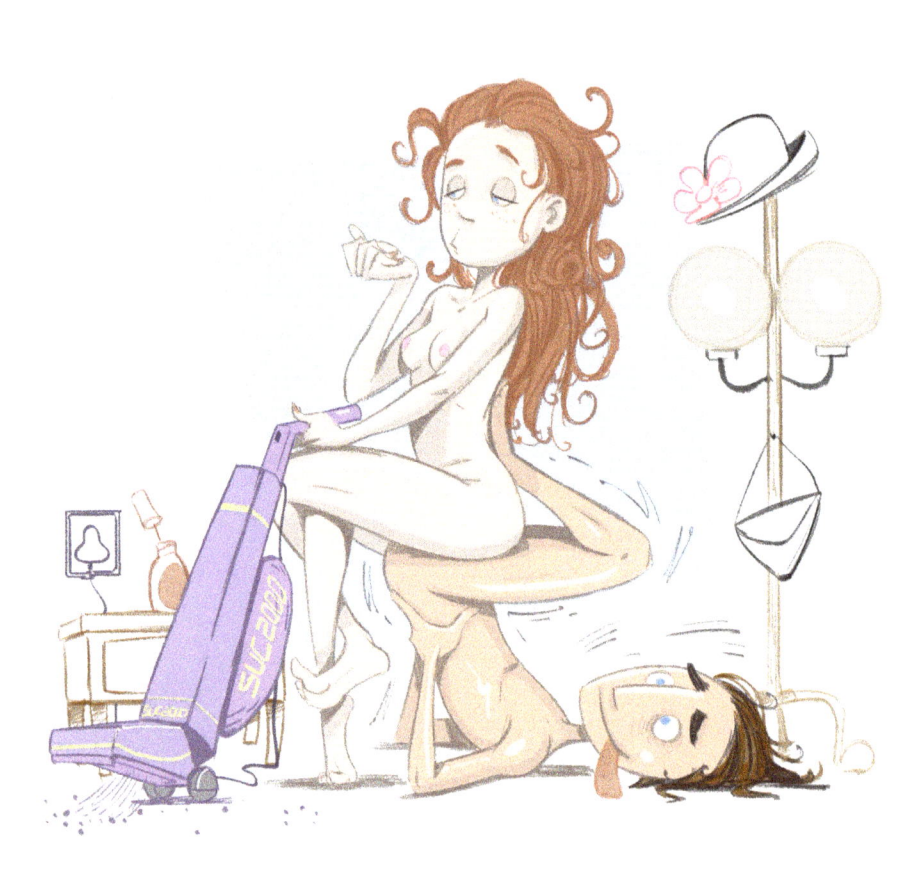

Vanilla is famed to increase arousal and sexual sensation.

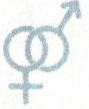

coconut pleasure

a little effort

\> 60 min

- 2 egg yolks
- 1¼ cup milk
- 2 vanilla pods, seeds removed
- ¾ cup cake flour, sifted
- 1 cup castor sugar
- 2 tsp baking powder
- ½ cup desiccated coconut
- ⅓ cup unsalted butter, melted
- knob of butter
- 2 handfuls fresh raspberries
- ¼ cup dark chocolate, finely grated

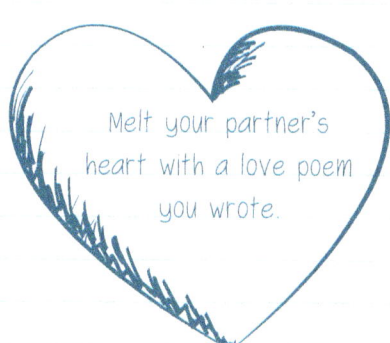

Melt your partner's heart with a love poem you wrote.

Whisk the eggs, milk and vanilla seeds together. In a large mixing bowl, combine the flour, sugar, baking powder and coconut. Make a well in the dry mixture, and pour the wet mixture and butter into the well. Mix together gently. Grease a loaf tin with butter and pour the mixture into the tin. Bake at 190°C for 45 minutes or until an inserted skewer comes out clean. Allow to cool and then remove from the tin. Sprinkle raspberries over and dust with the grated chocolate before serving.

Recommended:
Divert your attention to a Late Harvest Riesling.

The Party Quickie

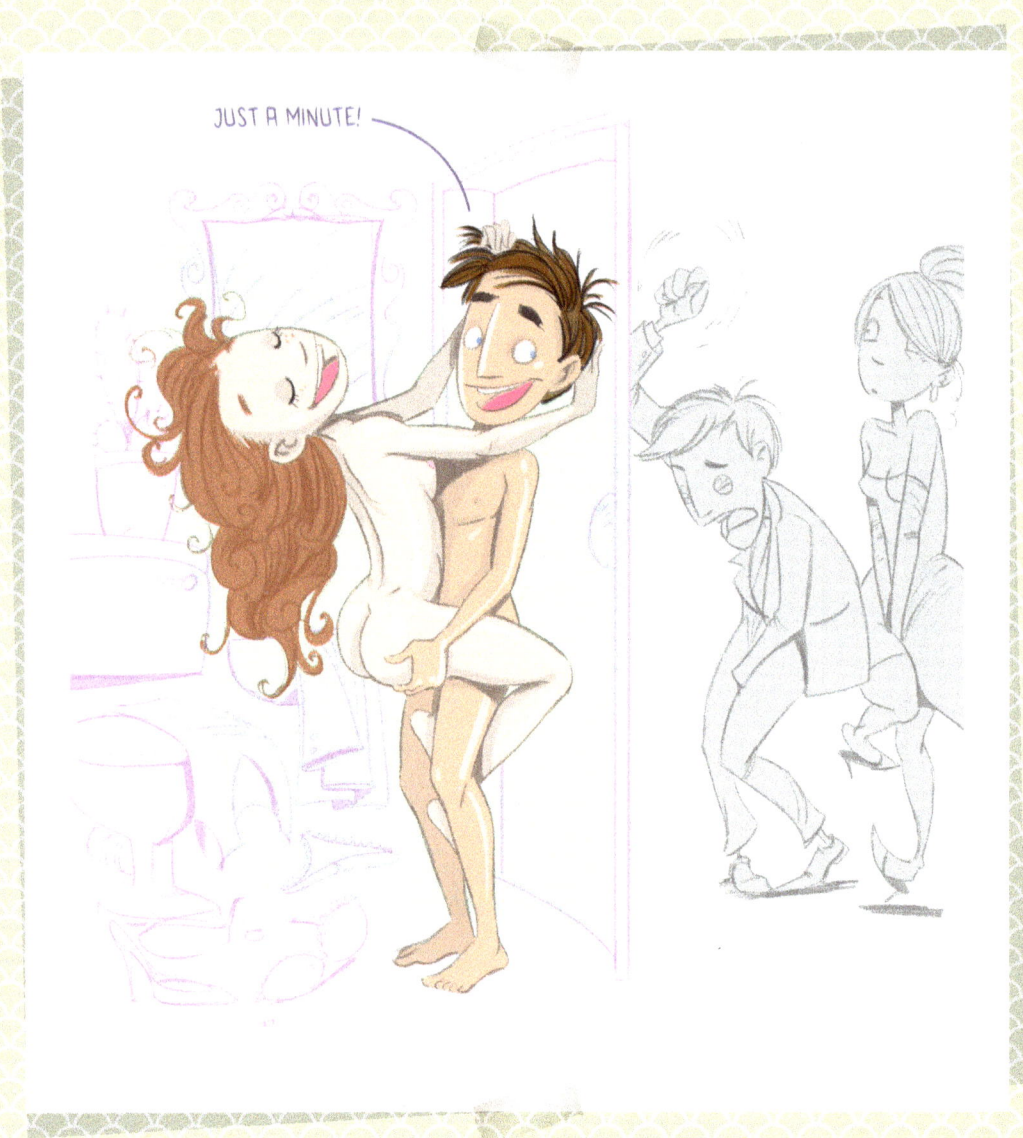

melt-in-mouth meringue

a little effort
\> 60 min

- 200g ginger biscuits
- 100g butter, melted
- 1 tin condensed milk
- ¼ cup lemon juice
- ¼ cup lime juice
- zest of 1 lemon
- zest of 1 lime
- 3 large eggs, separated and at room temperature
- ½ cup castor sugar
- 1 tsp castor sugar for dusting
- ¼ cup double-thick cream
- ½ cup tinned gooseberries, drained
- 2 sprigs of fresh lemon thyme

Crush the biscuits and mix well with the butter. Press a thin layer of biscuit mixture into a round baking tin so that the biscuit layer creeps up the sides. Put into the fridge for 30 minutes. In the meantime, whisk the condensed milk, lemon and lime juice, zest and egg yolks into a smooth mixture. Beat the egg-whites with an electric beater until you have firm and silky peaks. Turn the beater down to low and gradually add the sugar. Spread the egg-white mixture evenly over the condensed-milk mixture, and finish off with a dusting of sugar. Bake at 160°C for 25 minutes until the meringue is crisp. Turn off the oven and allow the lemon meringue pie to cool in the oven. Once cooled, place in the fridge until ready to serve. Serve with a dollop of cream, a few gooseberries and sprig of lemon thyme.

Recommended:
Quickly whip up this dessert so that you can get cracking with more important things. Take it with a shot of Limoncello.

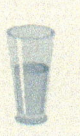

The Virgin

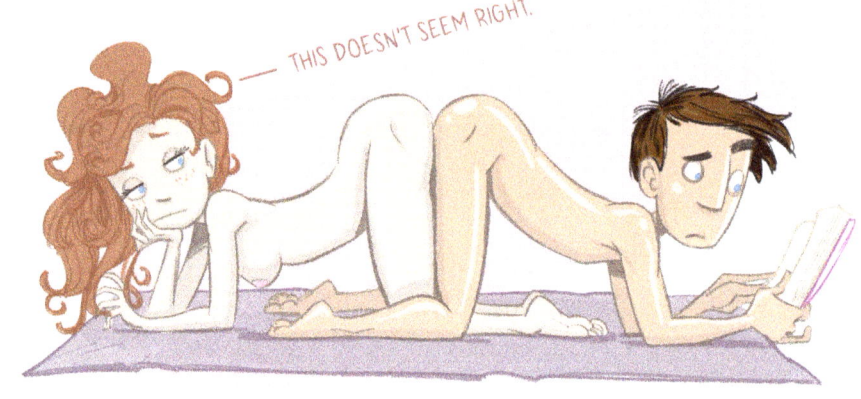

pop-the-cherry pie

a little effort
\> 60 min

- knob of butter
- 3 cups fresh cherries, whole and pitted
- 1 cup cake flour
- ½ cup castor sugar
- 2 vanilla pods, seeds removed
- pinch of salt
- 4 large eggs, at room temperature
- 2 tbsp amaretto liqueur
- 2 cups milk, boiled and cooled
- icing sugar for dusting
- ¼ cup almond flakes, lightly toasted

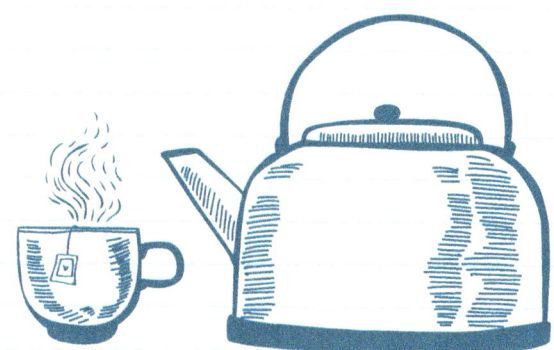

Use butter to grease a large pie dish and lay the cherries on the base. In a bowl add the flour, sugar, vanilla seeds and salt and mix. Add one egg at a time to the mixture, beating to combine. Gently fold in the amaretto and milk. Pour the mixture over the cherries and bake at 200°C for 40 minutes. Dust with icing sugar and a sprinkle of almonds.

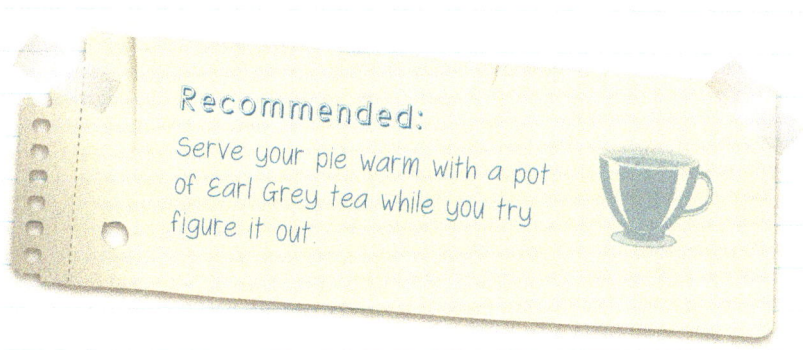

Recommended: Serve your pie warm with a pot of Earl Grey tea while you try figure it out.

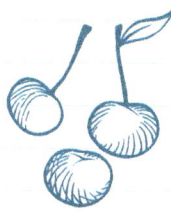

The Balancing Act

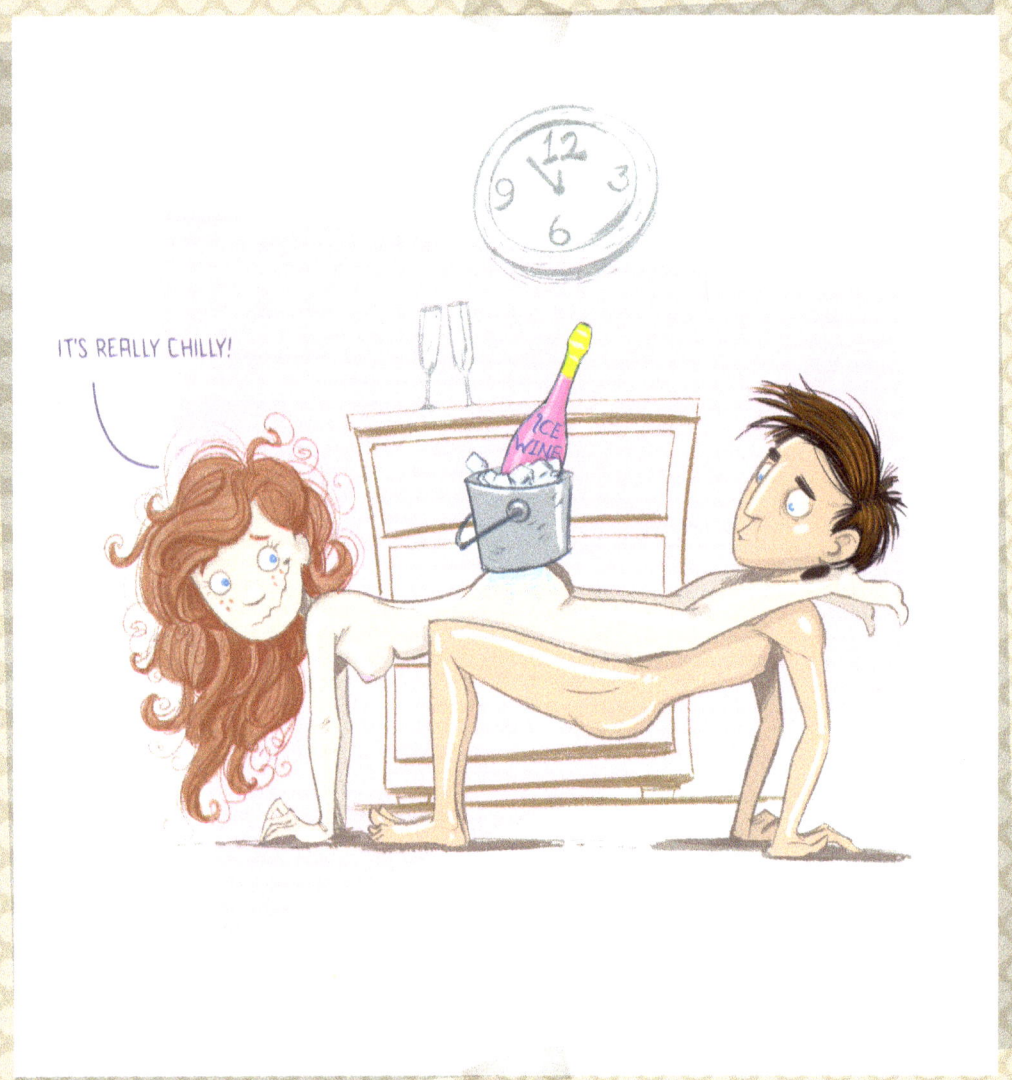

spicy custard

a little effort

\> 60 min

- 1¼ cup cream
- 2 cinnamon sticks
- 1 tsp ground nutmeg
- 2 tsp whole cloves
- 1 stick of lemon grass, sliced
- 1 cup water
- ½ cup palm sugar, grated
- 400ml coconut milk
- 3 eggs, lightly beaten
- 2 egg yolks, lightly beaten
- double-thick cream, for serving
- ¼ cup shredded coconut, lightly toasted, for serving
- 1 stick lemon grass, finely sliced, for garnishing

Put the cream, spices, lemon grass and water into a saucepan and bring to the simmer. Turn down the heat to the lowest setting and allow the spices to infuse the liquid for a few minutes. Turn the heat up to a low heat, and add the sugar and coconut milk, stirring until the sugar is dissolved. Remove from the heat. Whisk all the eggs together in a large bowl. Carefully pour the spiced mixture over the eggs and stir to combine. Strain the liquid through a sieve, and discard the whole pieces. Divide the custard mixture into ramekins and space out in a large roasting pan. Fill the pan with hot water until halfway up the ramekins and place in the oven for 45 minutes at 160°C. The custard is done when a skewer comes out clean and the mixture is still a little wobbly. Allow to cool and then place in the fridge to chill. Serve chilled with a dollop of cream, decorated with toasted coconut and a few lemon grass rings.

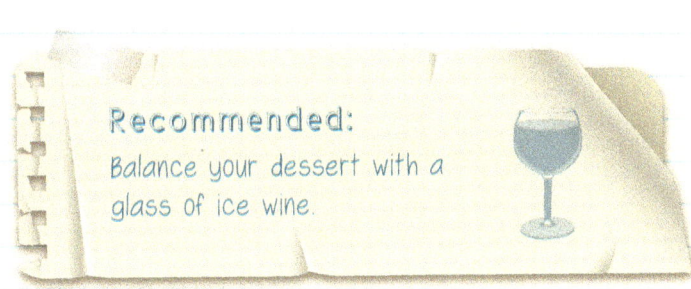

Recommended: Balance your dessert with a glass of ice wine.

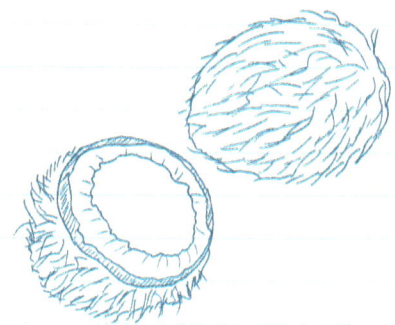

final thoughts

Unless it's a quickie take time to enjoy your food and each other.

www.ingramcontent.com/pod-product-compliance
Lightning Source LLC
Chambersburg PA
CBHW061753290426

44108CB00029B/2985